Praise for Dear

"This book provides so much guidance and practical tips for women who are about to go on this long and arduous course of treatment. We always wish and pray that no one ever has to go through this process, but I think the book will help patients immensely as they will have a general sense of what to expect. This is unlike any other book on cancer I have seen or read and it is refreshingly well written!"

A radiation oncologist

"I read her book in almost one sitting, it was so compelling and, through the excellence of her prose, was easy to read despite some rather technical details (all of which she explains in simple language) that she has obviously researched meticulously. Dear Cancer is full of information and hope that may be difficult to find from other sources. It is a great educational read that could change so many people's fears and perspectives of this disease, even if they've had no contact with it. The book is a treasure in which the reader laughs and cries with the author and I applaud that Ms. Marr can truly call herself a cancer survivor."

Susan Roebuck, writer and breast cancer survivor

Dear Cancer

Beating Triple Negative Breast Cancer

Ann Tracy Marr

Published by Ann Tracy Marr
anntracymarr@aol.com

Printed by CreateSpace

Copyright © 2015 by Ann Tracy Marr

First Edition: 2015
Printed in the United States of America

All rights reserved.
No part of this book may be reproduced or
transmitted in any form or by any electronic
or mechanical means, including photocopying, recording,
or by any information storage and
retrieval system without the written permission of
the publisher except where permitted by law.

Cover Art by Anthia Cumming. All rights reserved.

The drawing of a chest port was based on a graphic from
http://www.macmillan.org.uk.
Used by permission.

This is a work of non-fiction.
Names have been changed to protect privacy.

Available from Amazon.com
and other retail outlets.

ISBN-10: 1515250741
ISBN-13: 978-1515250746

This book is dedicated to my ideal husband.

The grayed words on the front cover are a listing of the medical tests and procedures the author experienced and research she undertook in the process of diagnosing and treating her triple negative breast tumors.

Contents

Diagnosis 1
    The Biopsy 5
    The MRI 18
    Definition of Triple Negative 23
Surgery 36
    The Pathology Report 52
Chemotherapy 58
    A Clinical Trial 63
    The Port 70
Chemotherapy Cycle 1 79
Chemotherapy Cycle 2 99
    Cancer Genetics 111
Chemotherapy Cycle 3 117
Chemotherapy Cycle 4 133
Chemotherapy Cycle 5 147
Chemotherapy Cycle 6 164
Radiation Therapy 176
    C Diff 193
    The Boost 204
Post-Treatment 211
    Physical Therapy and Yoga 212
    Cancer Antigens 218
Index to Side Effects and Symptoms
About the Author

Dear Reader,

I assume, since you picked up this book, that you or someone close to you has been diagnosed with breast cancer.

It isn't an easy time. If you are dealing with triple negative breast cancer, it gets harder. Triple negative is a deadly form of breast cancer. Information is not readily available and what one finds is discouraging. Because the cancer tends to be aggressive and there are fewer treatment options, those with a triple negative diagnosis often receive the maximum chemotherapy and the most radiation. What you don't get is a lot of hope.

I published this book to give you hope.

When I went through the ordeal, I was scared to death. I found that knowing things, having an idea what was going to happen, and learning about the different angles of the disease helped me through it all. You will read about what happened to me, plus get a lot of information on things I escaped. Your experience won't be exactly like mine, but it will give you an idea what to expect. And you will get lots of tips for dealing with your body.

I have no medical training; don't assume I know everything. If I missed something you run into, I suggest you ask your doctor for information.

My best advice is to keep your head up. I was told to be optimistic, which I found hard. I settled for determination. No way was cancer going to beat me. Whatever works for you—but don't let cancer beat you.

You have my prayers and best wishes,

Dear Cancer

Beating Triple Negative Breast Cancer

Diagnosis

Dear Cancer,

I just found out about you, that you have taken up residence in my left breast. I'm kicking you out, but until I know you are gone for good, I figure we might as well be friends. Well, not friends. Maybe acquaintances. Someone I wave to from the car as I drive by.

Drive by reminds me of shootings. That happens in Detroit; someone drives by a house and shoots a gun randomly (or not so randomly.) I don't know how many people die in those drive-by shootings because the news only tells us about the kids who get killed. Like that three year old baby, the one sleeping on the couch. My girls used to sleep on the couch. Chilling thought—if not for the grace of God, there goes one of my girls. Lots of things are chilling right now.

I vote to stop drive-by shootings, but let's have one more before we are done. How about I do a drive-by shooting on you, Cancer? I could go for that.

You picked a lousy time to announce your presence. I just got back from Katie's; it made sense to schedule my annual mammogram for after the trip to Sacramento. Since you were hiding in my breast, you know who Katie is. My eldest daughter, one of the lights of my life.

I am so darn proud of that girl—ahem, sorry to stomp on her ego. Twenty-something qualifies as a woman any way your life is lived, and Katie is doing well with hers.

She is an accountant; specifically, a government auditor. She lives about as far from her fond parents as she can get and still stay in the continental United States: California. She wants me to visit on a regular basis because auditors travel. Her cats go stir crazy when they go weeks on end seeing no one but a cat sitter. Having "Grandma" babysit the grandcats eases cats and Katie. One of the cats, Sibley, grew up in my house and heart. Arwen and I get along. Plus, I cook lots of casseroles. They get frozen in Katie-size portions and she doesn't have to worry about cooking.

The five years she has been in California has evolved a schedule. I am there sometimes in the spring, but certainly three times between July and Thanksgiving. We try to space the visits evenly to keep the cats from stressing out so badly they end up visiting the vet, which in turn stresses Katie.

I do it gladly. Katie means that much to me. *I like her a hell of a lot better than I like you, Cancer. Don't you dare screw this up.*

It was my second audit season visit. Most of the time I didn't have a car because it was shuffling Katie around the state doing those audits. I sat in her apartment, writing and playing games on my trusty laptop, loving cats, and filling the freezer.

I flew home after a pleasant two weeks in Sacramento, took a couple of days to decompress, and then scheduled errands.

Errand number one was at Cottage Hospital Woman's Center. I didn't want anything to do with the Center or their mammogram equipment. I had been there too often. Every year, or almost every year since I turned the ripe old age of thirty, I had been getting mammograms. Once, it had to be redone because they thought they saw something, but it was a false alarm. Occasionally, I missed a year and felt the weight of the world on my shoulders until I got the damn mammogram done.

It was cancer's fault. I had to be vigilant against it. It got into my mom when she was forty, made her miserable, helped break up her marriage, and ultimately killed her.

Mom had radiation to get rid of a tumor in her right breast. They overdid it and burned a hole in her chest that would not heal. Eventually, her chest got infected, the blood pressure between her heart and lungs increased, and her mitral valve gave way. Open heart surgery didn't have a chance against the infection. Mom was just a month under age 60 when she died. I had an 8½ month old baby Katie. She walked for the first time at Mom's funeral. I'd been bitter about that for more than twenty-five years.

Yes, cancer killed my mom.

Before it killed Mom, it killed her mom, my grandmother. It also killed her mom, my great-grandmother, according to her death certificate. And not too long ago it got into Mom's sister, but Mary Helen beat it. At least I think she did. Mary Helen died from a fall, not from rot in her breast. And years ago, in the 1920's, I think, cancer sneaked into Grandma's cousin. Lalie was a concert pianist and getting rid of cancer ruined her career. Surgeons in the 20's didn't have the advantage of today's breast cancer research; I am sure they just sliced and diced and Lalie got lucky. She lived to age 105.

Three generations of my mother's family suffered breast cancer. Because of them, I was considered high risk. I checked my genealogy; there weren't too many more women in the family; they lived to a decent age, but I don't know what killed them. For all I know, cancer attacked them also.

You are a scourge, Cancer.

Tuesday, September 27, 2011

Today was Errand Day. I took Martha (my younger daughter) to work, rushed to the Women's Center for my mammogram, spent money in stores, and stopped at Janet's Lunch to eat. I didn't do as many errands as I should. My heart wasn't in it because the mammogram procedure depresses me.

The Woman's Center is set up with an eye to detail. It has to be one of the nicest places to have a mammogram done and I wanted out of there in the worst way. They treat you like a Waterford crystal queen. No rough moves so you don't chip. When you sign in, they automatically give you a ticket to pay for parking. No questions asked and the ticket is good for the whole day, so you can go shopping on The Hill. That's the pricey shopping district for the rich suburbs of Grosse Pointe. Grosse Pointe as in the residences of Fords and Fishers, the auto heroes of Detroit. Doctors, lawyers, rich people, live in Grosse Pointe. As do I, and we are far from rich. We cling to the incredible shrinking middle class; I don't shop on The Hill.

The Woman's Center receptionists are pleasant—no snarly dragons here. Today's newspaper is available. The chairs in the waiting room are comfortable, but that doesn't matter because you don't spend a lot of time on them. You are in and out with no fuss. At least that was what always happened to me.

The dressing room has two doors—the one you enter from the hall locks, so your purse is safe while your breast is being pummeled by the mammogram machine. The other door goes into the X-ray room. The temperature is balmy; the technician is as nice as the receptionist. She apologizes for squeezing your breast into a pancake and she sounds like she might mean it. She is efficient. The whole procedure is as nice as it can get.

The lady took my pictures and I left.

Monday, October 3, 2011

You messed up my day, Cancer. The Woman's Center called. I was back for more tests, this time an ultrasound of two areas in my left breast. The receptionist didn't chat much. She handed me over to the lions for mauling.

I was ushered to the dressing room because they wanted a couple more mammograms. Too bad there isn't a lock on both doors—I could have barricaded myself in until someone admitted it was an elaborate joke. Better sadistic jokes than the possibility of cancer.

Then came the ultrasound. The ultrasound technician lion I was thrown to was a young woman—at least younger than I. The ultrasound was like any medical procedure. I reclined on the table while she ran the wand over my breast on the outside side and slightly below. The gel was exactly body temperature so I couldn't feel it on my skin. She took some pictures and was done.

The rubbing was relentless, so my breast was a little sore. The technician and the radiologist harped at each other; was the one area at four or five? And the other; was it one or two? They settled between four and five and between one and two. I imagined a clock face and tried to reconcile it with where the ultrasound wand dug.

It appeared that if it was anything, I caught it early. The radiologist would look the pictures over and they would call.

The coordinator-head nurse-consultant—well, I don't know what her title was, but her name was Pat—took me into her office for some literature and information. Her motherly, comforting attitude grated on my nerves. I escaped, ran two errands, ate at Janet's, and went home. Enough was enough.

Tuesday, October 4, 2011

The Woman's Center called. They wanted to do a biopsy. Oh, hell. I couldn't need a biopsy; that meant it might be cancer. Forget family history. I didn't want to deal with it.

I told Rick. He didn't get it, I don't think. This was not a surprise; my husband was under tremendous stress at work. Sometimes things went over his head. Still, he was extra sweet. I didn't talk; I didn't really want to discuss it. It made it more real.

Sweet is Rick's usual state. I like macho-macho men in romances, but in real life, I would cost a pushy, arrogant alpha male in the jaw the minute he started ordering me around. I certainly didn't marry one. My husband is more like Ward Cleaver (remember Leave It To Beaver?) He goes to work, comes home and doesn't complain if dinner isn't on the table. He loves his kids and has trouble criticizing them. He loves his wife (me!) and doesn't fool around behind her back. He is easy to live with, easy to get along with, and easy to love. Rick is a constant plus in an often negative world.

Martha's response (more about this angel later) was matter-of-fact. She was too absorbed in learning how to live her adult life to be concerned with mine. Katie called, so I told her. I don't think it sank in there either.

The Biopsy

Wednesday, October 5, 2011

There I was, in a maroon hospital gown, crossing the hall of the Woman's Center because the ultrasound room is across the hall from the dressing room. The hall was deserted. Using ESP, I knew the women working there made sure it was empty of people so I wouldn't be embarrassed being seen in that awful hospital gown. Maybe their other clients didn't want the reminder that this nasty thing called breast cancer does happen. Or maybe they were just protecting my privacy so no one knew it was me facing the ax.

Hey, Cancer, do you hang out at the Woman's Center to see the reactions of those you torment? I'm younger than most of the females I saw there; is that why you picked on me? Am I supposed to be more surprised than these old ladies at the threat of something foreign growing in me? Not hardly. Since I was twelve, when Mom had to deal with you, I trained myself for your emergence. It is better to be prepared than shocked.

I'll let you know when I figure out if I am shocked or fatalistic.

Was I was scared? Nervous, yes. Scared? Well, I didn't run screaming from the room. If I paid attention, I had butterflies in my stomach. If I ignored them, they weren't there. Let's forget that my hands were shaking.

I was on the same hospital bed as I was for the ultrasound. It was narrow, with wheels, so if I went Code Red or whatever, they could wheel me through the halls to the Emergency Room at the back of the building. Oh, really. We don't need high drama. Let's just get this done with. It was a party with the technician, the radiologist and Pat. Yes, Pat was there.

It was the same radiologist as did the ultrasound. This time, I looked at his face. His young face. It figured. I noticed a couple of years ago that I had gotten older than the people who manage my illnesses. It didn't matter except I was no longer intimidated by them. I was this guy's equal even though he was going to stick a big needle into my breast and feed another thing through that to break off bits of the suspicious stuff to look at.

He was a doctor and it was a biopsy, as simple as that.

It made me glad that I had borne two children, undergone a D&C for a failed pregnancy, had Paps and pelvic exams, etc. Somewhere in all those medical procedures, I lost the concept of modesty around doctors. Who cared that I was lying on a table with my boob staring at this guy's face? I couldn't imagine him going home to his wife and saying, "I worked on this woman today. You should have seen..."

I didn't feel embarrassed. I couldn't remember his name, and I didn't care about his point of view.

First, the radiologist marked my left breast with a big blue slash on top. Not X marks the spot, but a slash. We had an enlightening discussion of how some surgeons mark the pertinent part of a pair with an X to indicate that "this one counts," and others do the opposite. Doctors are as bad as the computer industry, which can't agree on where the Delete key belongs on a keyboard. Standardization is good. They should teach it in medical school or send new doctors to do a six week internship with pirates.

My arm went above my head, out of the way, and he washed me with an alcohol liquid. It was cool and refreshing on a warm day. Then they draped blue paper pads over me. One flopped in my face, but that didn't matter. I was supposed to have my head to the side. Gee, I got to watch the ultrasound monitor.

The technician ran the wand over my breast. She found the first area quickly, so the thing about four and five o'clock was useful. She pointed it out. It looked like a long piece of spaghetti with a dark spot or hole in it. Not big, not impressive. I hoped it was as insignificant as it looked.

I felt the first pinch of the needle that numbed my breast. Then I felt something else and the radiologist assured me it was okay to react. A flinch would tell him there was another nerve to be pacified. If I'd been in one of those moods, I would have assured him that I lived through Vietnam War protests. Pacification was for war hawks, not nerves. I really didn't feel anything else except light pressure here and there.

I let them do their thing, and no, I didn't watch the ultrasound monitor after that first view. I did talk; Coordinator Pat kept me going as a distraction. I talked too much and didn't care.

There was a series of sharp sounds. I jumped when I first heard it; the radiologist asked if I felt something. I'm not sure if I told him no. I did say, "You shot me." It wasn't a drive-by shooting; the shooting was the snipping of suspicious stuff. By the time he was done with the second area, the one between one and two, I hardly twitched at the sound. I should have asked him to warn me before the sound; then I might not have flinched at all. But I wasn't thinking. He snipped more from the first area than the second.

With the first area, the radiologist told me he got very good samples. How could he tell? Breast fat floats in the solution they dump it into and my samples sank like stones. I felt comforted, but really, I didn't know that I should. It'd have been better if my suspicious areas were merely dark colored breast fat. Fat with freckles? They should float on their backs and sip tequila.

Then I got presents. I was gifted with the information that I had a microcalcification (a tiny spot of calcium. A cluster can indicate the presence of cancer, but I was told a calcification, not a cluster,) and two areas that were so small they hadn't had time to form a mass. I also got two tiny titanium markers shot into the suspicious spots, not even big enough to set off the security scanners at the airport. If the areas were okay, those markers would sit there the rest of my life. If not, they were X marks the spot for surgery.

I was more interested in the vision of setting off the scanner at the airport. The next time I flew to see Katie, I'd get to the airport five minutes earlier, just in case.

I got out of the Woman's Center with two band-aids, two ice packs (for swelling,) two titanium markers, and one parking ticket pass. I was surprised how unsteady on my feet I was. The stupid butterflies kept coming back, and every once in a while, I felt like crying. I pampered myself the rest of the day; in other words, I didn't do anything productive.

The ice packs were useful for a while, and then they were a nuisance.

Martha, Daughter #2, who graduated from college after the economy fell apart, was shafted by Obama, or Bush, or Wall Street, or whoever or whatever was responsible for the problems in the country. There weren't any jobs, there was nowhere for her to go. So she came home and took a series of part-time jobs. Determined to get into her chosen field, she sent out resume after resume. She became an intern for a local congressman. As her hours with his office increased, she dropped part-time jobs. Now, she was a staffer in the re-election campaign office.

Martha was the shocker. Before, she was a typical busy, never-home daughter. When she heard about the biopsy, she rallied to the cause. Became supportive. Did things without being asked. Made life easier for me.

Cancer, go away and let me enjoy Martha's company. She'll be gone soon enough. With my luck, she'll be on the East Coast while her sister is on the West Coast and their dad and I are stuck in the Midwest.

Thursday, October 6, 2011

I still felt shaky.

I made an appointment for Monday at the doctor's office to find out the results of the biopsy. My regular doctor, Dr. Sanatio, was out of the office for a week, so I couldn't see him. Damn, I'd rather see Dr. Sanatio. He'd give me more and better information than anyone else. Still, I was not waiting an extra week for him to return. I'd see some doctor I never saw before and find out if I had cancer.

I was doing my best not to worry. I floated along, doing my work, and then I'd stop and think. I was worried.

My breast was still a little sore. If I got up and moved around, I felt it. Funny, I didn't usually notice that my breasts bounced when I walked.

I called Blue Cross to find out if I could get the genetic test for cancer. It might not make any difference for me, but I had two daughters who might care. Not to mention four cousins, and four girls in the next generation. No, it couldn't be authorized, not without a diagnosis.

I don't want to die. I don't want to have cancer. I don't want to have surgery. Go away, Cancer. Don't happen.

Friday, October 7, 2011

I recovered my equilibrium. I wasn't happy, but I could deal with whatever came.

Monday, October 10, 2011

I was due at the doctor at 2:45. I was antsy. I wanted to know, I wanted to know. I wasn't scared. I was nervous. Martha was home because the office was closed for Columbus Day. Bless her, she asked if I wanted her to come. Yes, I did. I'm not stupid. If I got bad news, I might need her to drive.

The Detroit Lions were 5-0 for the season. That hadn't happened since 1956, the year I was born. Good for them. The Detroit Tigers were fighting to get to the World Series. Good luck to them. It was one of those perfect fall days—warm, sunny, absolutely perfect—and I didn't enjoy it. Not one bit. I felt cheated. I never did care much about sports and I was too preoccupied to enjoy nice weather.

Nothing like getting there early. Early enough for the receptionist to go over the insurance. It was new with Rick's new job and scrambled. We had Blue Cross, only it used to be Anthem Blue Cross and it turned into Empire Blue Cross. The card said that if you're in California, bill Anthem. If you are anywhere else, bill Empire. The office wanted to bill Anthem. I got it straightened out, which kept my mind busy. My mind needed to be busy.

Then the doctor came to the exam room. She was pretty, with long dark hair that curled just enough. Dimly, I appreciated this girl's looks. And wouldn't you know, she wasn't just younger, she looked young enough to be Martha. As usual, I couldn't remember her name. She had papers in her hand. The biopsy report, I was sure.

Just give it to me.

I didn't need her name. I didn't need her bedside manner either. She gave me this intent look as she asked why I was there. I can be blunt; I told her I was there to find out if I had cancer or not. She couldn't be equally blunt. She wanted to go through the report bit by bit. I reined in my impatience. It took her a while to get to the fact that I had cancer.

The biopsy was positive.

I let her blather—Martha would pay attention to what she said—cover the bases. Then I pulled myself together and told the doctor that I was going to go home and get on the Internet—pull out all the information I could find. She was horrified. Don't do that! Chat rooms wouldn't give me accurate information. No, but the Mayo Clinic would.

Then, the girl slipped. Looking properly distressed, she mentioned "advanced state." It slammed into me. It slammed into Martha too. But she had realized her mistake; we couldn't get any more information out of her. She had set up an appointment for Wednesday with the oncologist. Wait and talk to him; he would give me all the information I wanted. Then, realizing that I really did intend to go home and go on the Internet, she volunteered to print out some information.

So Martha and I sat in the room forever, it seemed. The doctor was slow doing her printing. Maybe she had to check with someone as to what she should print, but I thought she was giving me time to break down and time for Martha to put me back together. Instead, we laid plans. I wanted food and a rum and Coke. Martha needed food.

Finally we escaped with the first page of the biopsy report and a handful of informational pages. We got the hell out of there. I was proud that I only choked up twice. My mom, with her very English proper behavior code, would have been proud of my stiff upper lip.

Yes, Martha heard it too. What did that doctor mean, "advanced state"?

We went to Little Tony's, a bar with excellent burgers and Bacardi.

Bless my girl; she was up to the challenge. Rather than getting all misty eyed and emotional, Martha sat next to me in the booth and we devoured the papers page by page. The biopsy report was succinct. I had a left breast mass at 1-2 o'clock which was part of a benign cyst wall. Benign. Not cancer.

I had a left breast mass 4-5 o'clock position that was invasive ductal carcinoma.

That is you, Cancer, damn you. Lousy way to introduce yourself. Why can't you be simple? Estrogen receptor was negative. Progesterone receptor was negative. Neither of us had a clue what that meant.

That's what the Internet was for: cold hard facts. I wished the doctor had given us the other pages of the report; what did they say? The sinking feeling in my gut said I needed to learn as much about cancer as I could, but I had to wait until Wednesday to find out more.

The pages that took so long printing were from MD Consult, an Internet site. Thank God, information to sink my teeth into. The topic was Breast Cancer; there was a Summary, Synonyms, Immediate action, Urgent action, and Key points, followed by three pages of background going over causes, risk factors, statistics and demographics. I read it all, passing pages to Martha as I finished so she could read them. It was disappointing. There was nothing to sink my teeth into. That doctor thought she could pacify me with this non-technical, basic stuff and keep me away from the Internet.

No, I wanted real information—what was I facing? What to do to save my life?

Life went on, at least for now. I had a computer to pick up. Holly probably had a virus; I'd take it home and fix it. That is one of my jobs, fixing computers. No employees, just little old me. Way back when, I added writing to my list of things to do. The first book went unpublished. It was a thoroughly researched, written from the heart recounting of the story of my great-great-grandmother's two brothers, the ones who were railroaded into prison in the 1880's. I think it's a good book. Martha thinks it's my best book, but I couldn't get anyone interested in it. Oh, well, I wrote and published three romances. The fourth book was on the editor's desk, and a couple of unfinished manuscripts were on my hard drive.

Now I was writing this diary. If nothing else, it was therapy. Writing focused my brain. It fulfilled a need. If nothing else ever got published, I would still write.

Martha and I got home sometime before 5 o'clock, a time I would forever after associate with cancer. It was between 4 and 5 o'clock, you know. Bad me, I ignored Holly's computer and went on the Internet and yes, the Mayo Clinic came through for me. Lots of other sites cooperated also.

Invasive ductal carcinoma is cancer that is born in a milk duct. If the cancer sits in the duct, not figuring out how to break free and wander around, it is called in situ, nicknamed DCIS, and is much less deadly. It isn't going to spread. If the tumor manages to pickaxe through the duct wall and make a bid for freedom (spread or metastasize,) it is plain old invasive ductal carcinoma, the most frequently diagnosed breast cancer, and the second most common cause of cancer death. Okay, I was as common as dirt.

Martha texted her sister and told her. I was glad and mad. I wanted to tell Katie myself, but not until I had something solid to report—like what was going to happen. Katie had enough to do without fretting about me.

I called her. The poor girl was so swamped that for the first time ever, she wasn't prepared for the audit. The county wasn't ready either, so Katie was able to do the planning today. My call interrupted; she had a pile of things to do. No, a government auditor doesn't work 9 to 5, not during audit season. She works from eyelids open to eyelids closed. I could tell she relegated me to the back of her mind; all she wanted to know was that I was still coming to Sac.

Yes, I was supposed to fly to Sacramento in two weeks. I planned to stay two weeks, take care of the cats and fill Katie's freezer with meals. Please, God, let me go to Sacramento. I wanted to see my Katie.

I didn't know if I was being unrealistic, but right then I was irritated with this cancer thing. It was going to get in the way of doing what I wanted to do. I didn't want to bother with it.

Wait, not done with info dumping.

The only other information I had was that my cancer was Estrogen receptor negative and Progesterone receptor negative. That is not so common. More commonly, the receptors are positive, meaning the cancer is influenced by hormones. Give the tumor a shot of hormones and it picks up weights and grows muscle.

If I had known that my cancer was going to ignore hormones, I would have done hormone replacement therapy when I went through menopause. Because of my family's breast cancer history, I couldn't take hormones. They can cause cancer. That is the sort of situation the word irony was invented to handle.

I forgot to cook dinner; I forgot that Holly's computer was on the floor, begging for tests. I could remember that I was Estrogen and Progesterone receptor negative. I just wasn't sure what it meant for me. I remembered the computer after dinner, which Martha cooked. I stayed up until 3 am working on the machine. It was really sick. I buried my worry with work.

Tuesday, October 11, 2011

I still have the marks from my first battle with you, Cancer: two bruises from the biopsy. They don't show, they don't hurt. What does hurt is the mess one of the band-aids made on the side of my breast. The skin there is more sensitive; the band-aid pulled from the edge and gave me what looks and feels like a rug burn. A bad rug burn. It scabbed over, but it stings.

If that is the worst you do to me, it will be a miracle. Yes, I know you are a nasty son of a bitch. You're going to give me more pain, both mental and physical. But you are not going to win, Mr. Cancer. I am.

I called and told Holly that I was still working on her computer. Even if I had started working on it the moment I got home yesterday, it still wouldn't go back to her. There was a nasty, nasty something somewhere on her hard drive. Sometimes you admit defeat and wipe the computer clean and start over, but that was not an option with this one. It had business specific programs that would be a nightmare to reload, plus I would be sure to lose valuable data in those programs. I had to dig to find the problem. But Holly kept me occupied. Lots better than sitting around stewing.

I spent the day rolling my chair back and forth between Holly's computer and mine. Holly's ran antivirus and anti-malware programs all day, with a break once for Chkdsk to verify that the hard drive was not scrambled. My computer ran the Internet and Microsoft Word. I was searching for information about Invasive Ductal Carcinoma & Co., writing this diary, and when I couldn't stand it anymore, playing Pogo.

Pogo is a games website. Mother may I? Sometimes I was there too much, but often, I was there to clear my brain. Writing, I discovered that playing Pogo allowed my subconscious to figure out plot twists. I would work on a scene, type like mad, and suddenly "run dry," as in I just couldn't write any more. It was not that I didn't know where the scene was heading. I already knew that. It was the details that tied the scene to the rest of the story that snarled. I'd consciously try to work out a pesky wrinkle, but sometimes that wasn't enough. My subconscious wanted to get involved and I didn't have control over it. Mindless distraction, like playing Pogo, did the trick.

I ignored my email. There was plenty there, but not today. I wrote my diary until I had nothing further to say and started a heavy duty Pogo session. It was distraction. I was not writing anything that required plotting; I was recording events. And I didn't want to record anymore. I wanted to forget.

I didn't have enough information to research the Internet. I needed to know what stage I was. How big was the tumor? How advanced was it? Did the radiologist lie when he said it was so small it hadn't formed a mass? Was the girl doctor insane when she said, "Advanced state?"

I only knew I would have either a lumpectomy or a mastectomy. If it was lumpectomy, they take a melon baller and dig out the cancer. If it was mastectomy, they cut off my breast. They cut off my mother's breast. They also took out the lymph nodes under her arm and burned her up with radiation. I saw Mom's chest; it wasn't a pretty sight. God, I didn't want to do that to myself.

Wednesday, October 12, 2011

Today I would find out if I was likely to die from cancer.

Holly had her computer back. Everything worked except her antivirus. I put another antivirus program on at 1 am and went to bed at 2.

I drove Martha to work, visited Holly, and went to Janet's for breakfast. Janet's Lunch, to be precise. It is a 1940's era diner, hardly updated, with a long counter in a U. It's the same countertop my aunt had on her kitchen table in the 1960's, gray and white streaked linoleum. I usually sat at the top of the right side of the U where I could watch the cook. I don't like cooking myself, but I enjoy watching someone else do the work.

All morning I had a knot in my stomach.

If Monday's weather was great, today's was typical. Not warm, but not cold yet. I couldn't decide if I should keep my sweater on or not, but the drizzling rain said to wear it. There was no incentive to do anything remotely useful. I hung out at Janet's until I had to pick up Martha.

She was hungry; I took my twenty-some-year-old baby to McDonald's and bought her a Cheeseburger Happy Meal. Then we drove to the Henry Ford Health System office where the oncologist would put me out of my misery.

The knot was still in my stomach.

We timed it perfectly and didn't sit long in the waiting room.

I appreciated the nurse's attitude, efficient but compassionate. Not cloying or pitying. She weighed me, never a happy prospect, then put me and Martha in a room. I had to change into another hospital gown, but this one needed to go in the trash. It had outlived its usefulness. What the hay, the economy was tough all over. If Henry Ford had to save money by using thin, limp hospital gowns, I could live with it. And I meant that literally. I was alive to put up with things.

Then the doctor came in. Happiness at last, he was older than I. Emotionally, I could look up to him as a father figure. With cancer, I think I preferred authority ordering me around. But Dr. Chirurgus was not the hardnosed boss demanding excellence; he was the fatherly type. I didn't have to sit on the exam table. He wanted me to pull my chair up next to his to talk. Martha too—she wasn't excluded.

And the information poured out.

The radiologist was correct. My tumor was 6x7x4 millimeters. (Bad info here to be explained later.) Roughly oval. If it was any smaller, they probably wouldn't have seen it on the mammogram. He checked last year's mammogram; it wasn't there then. Because it was so small, there was little or no chance it had spread to my lymph nodes; they just don't start moving around at that size.

There was a punctate calcification (punctate means it isn't smooth, it is pock marked; calcification means a tiny bit of calcium) in the middle of the tumor, but he didn't think anything of it.

The tumor was not responsive to estrogen or progesterone. It was moderately differentiated, as in the cells didn't look normal, but they were not wildly weird either. If only I had known what it all meant! I didn't ask.

Dr. Chirurgus had the next several months planned for me. First, I needed to go downstairs and have a blood test to check my kidney function. Once the results showed up on the computer, the Radiology Department would schedule a MRI. The MRI would look for evidence of tumors in my breasts that the mammogram missed.

If the MRI found something more, I would have a mastectomy. But if it didn't—he was very optimistic on this—I would have a lumpectomy with wire localization, a sentinel biopsy of lymph nodes under my arm, and radiation therapy for six weeks. He left the idea of chemotherapy up in the air. I would not have hormonal therapy because my tumor would ignore it.

Let's translate to make sure I got it all straight. A lumpectomy is when they put me to sleep and cut a slit in my breast (it would look something like a smiley face to follow the natural curve of my breast) and burrow in to cut out the tumor. Dr. Chirurgus would remove roughly a one inch ball, doing his best to get all of the cancer. My breast might end up a little smaller, but it should look okay.

The wire localization is done before the surgery. While I was awake, they would numb my breast and shove guide wires in to do what else but

X marks the spot. He would inject blue dye and a radioactive substance in next to the tumor and watch to see where it all went. The first lymph node the junk got to was called the Sentinel node. That was the node he would take out and check for cancer cells. If there weren't any, I could jump for joy because the cancer had not metastasized.

We didn't discuss what happened if they found cancer in the node. We were not borrowing a crutch. (If there is cancer in a lymph node, everything jumps up. That means the cancer spread.)

We didn't spend a lot of time talking about radiation therapy. I asked if my hair would fall out—no, it wouldn't—enough.

Every question I asked, the nurse or the doctor handed me a piece of paper or a booklet. Good—that was more information to go through. I wanted information—I wanted details—I wanted to KNOW. If I didn't beat cancer, it wouldn't be from ignorance.

There was a breast cancer clinic the following week. I'd talk to oncologists, surgeons, everyone. I could get a second opinion. Sounded like the smart thing to do.

And I could go to Sacramento.

Leaving the doctor's office felt like escape from Alcatraz. Martha and I planned a celebration. Not to celebrate cancer, but to rejoice that the tumor was so damn small and my chances sounded so good. Rick would be home late, so we stopped at a deli and bought sandwiches and soup for dinner. And five desserts for the three of us. It cost a fortune but it was a good deli.

Thursday, October 13, 2011

I still felt giddy. It was relief, plain and simple. The radiologist didn't lie to me; the oncologist was optimistic. The stupid cancer was tiny, almost insignificant.

No, it wasn't insignificant. More research on the Internet told me that. The tumor was not responsive to hormones so that knocked out a chunk of treatment. It classified my cancer as harder to cure. All sorts of pills help to starve a tumor that responds to hormones. They call it hormonal therapy. The cancers that most often are influenced by hormones are breast, prostate, ovarian and endometrial. What hormones make the cancer happy? Estrogen, progesterone, and androgen get star billing.

What do the doctors do if your tumor responds to those hormones? Well, they might want to remove your ovaries, the primary producers of estrogen and progesterone. They might give you medications to suppress the production of hormones or have you undergo radiation.

After treatment, provided the tumor is eliminated, they want to do more to prevent the cancer from coming back. The more is hormonal medication. Pop pills or get injections to keep cancer from bouncing back. The medicines do different things, work different ways, but are effective against hormone hungry cancer.

One of the biggies, Tamoxifen, is a pill that you take every day for five years—it stops cancer from gorging on estrogen. You have to take it every day—don't forget!—and have to take it for the full five years if you want the benefit of staving off cancer for at least ten more years. It has side effects, such as increased risk for blood clots and endometrial (uterine) cancer, and menopausal symptoms. Aromatase inhibitors stop the aromatase enzyme from producing estrogen.

Side effects include higher blood cholesterol levels, bone thinning, and joint pain. Other medications decrease the amount of hormones produced in your body by messing up the signals the brain sends out. Look for more side effects from them.

I wasn't thrilled with the idea of side effects, but I would have loved having pills available to fight my cancer.

I hadn't discussed it with the doctor, but I was pretty sure that lack of further treatment options meant that he had to be sure to dig all of the tumor out. I didn't want cancer to come back.

Another danger involved Her-2/neu (it stands for human epidermal growth factor receptor.) My pathology report didn't say what mine was. The test had been ordered and was pending. I wasn't sure what Her-2/neu meant.

And what was the triple negative type of tumor and why was it bad? It is the most dangerous type of breast cancer, but again, I didn't know what it was—or if I had it. I felt slap-happy, but deep inside, the knot was waiting to jump back into my stomach.

It was time to get the family in the loop. I emailed basic info to relatives and told them I would keep them informed.

Then, like a responsible adult (one who has suffered through insurance mix-ups too often,) I called the member phone number on my Blue Cross card. Amazingly, it was not hard to find a real, live person, and that person was actually helpful.

I told Blue Cross lady that I had been diagnosed with breast cancer and I didn't even know what the co-pay was for office visits. After all, the insurance went into effect August 1 when the company Rick works for changed and I hadn't been sick.

Right off the bat, she gave me good news. There was no co-pay for office visits. I could see Dr. Sanatio all I wanted and I wouldn't be billed. Hip hip hooray. But there was a 25% co-pay for visits to specialists like oncologists—the doctor who was going to be my best friend by Christmas.

The maximum we had to pay was $4,270 for the year. Of course, our year started August 1 and went to December 31 and any amount we paid to the old Blue Cross didn't count. Old employer, old Blue Cross. New employer, new Blue Cross. We owed $90 for the biopsy. $90 for the simplest step in dealing with cancer suggested that $4,270 was going to come hard and fast. Our savings account was not that big. If I was really stupid, I would wait until January to do something about the cancer.

No, I was not that stupid. When my mother was diagnosed with breast cancer, treatment was delayed because my self-employed father had cancelled our health insurance. She had to wait until he found the money for insurance. Big help—it was a pre-existing condition and... I don't know details. All I know is she had to wait and the cancer was in her lymph nodes.

You don't wait.

After I talked and talked and talked with the Blue Cross lady, I made another call to check that I was signed up for the next step in my whirlwind tour of Cancerland: the Breast Cancer Clinic, a program put together by Henry Ford Health System. Next Thursday, starting at 8 am, Rick and I would spend up to five hours at Henry Ford Hospital, meeting the doctors who would beat up my cancer.

We could get questions answered. I had several:
- Radiation therapy can damage the heart. What do we do about that, other than not have radiation therapy, which I fully intended to have?
- Her-2/neu—was it positive or negative? What did it mean?
- Were there more details available from Pathology? I wanted every scrap.
- How many breast cancer surgeries were performed at the hospital every year and how many did my doctor do—I should get the dull statistics that told me if Dr. Chirurgus was competent or if I should run screaming elsewhere.
- Considering that my tumor was hormone negative, should I have a mastectomy rather than a lumpectomy? Not that I wanted my breast sliced off, but what was the reasoning for not going that route?
- What were the results of the MRI (the one I would have on Saturday?)
- The care and feeding of my queenly self after surgery.

- The care and feeding of my still queenly self during and after radiation therapy. I had not even asked where the radiation therapy was done. Should I get over the hurdle of surgery first?

I didn't have my questions in any logical order and Rick was sure to add to them.

Internet research turned up the results of a few studies done on breast cancer patients. Curiously, joining a support group does not seem to affect survival rates, but encouragement from family and friends does. Survival rates go up if your family and friends remain positive. Over dinner, I demanded that my family be fully supportive until this was over and done with—or else. As if I needed to say it.

I have a good family, a loving family.

Friday, October 14, 2011

This was the first normal day all week. No doctor appointments. I was so tired, I sat in front of the TV and fell asleep in the afternoon. I only did that when I was sick. What would make me think I was sick?

I had no patience for things that didn't go right the first time. I had to burn a CD; when the CD drive refused to recognize a blank disk, I walked away. Rick would do it.

But my tumor had not metastasized. Cancers that spread are much more dangerous. Harder to get rid of, more capable of killing you. Most of the people who die from triple negative breast cancer die because it has metastasized. If it is going to spread, breast cancer usually heads for lymph nodes, bones, lungs, liver or brain. If it reaches the lymph nodes, that is considered the most treatable metastasis.

Don't despair if your cancer has spread. Despair doesn't help. Think positive (studies have shown that your state of mind does affect the outcome of treatment.) Turn into an Amazon warrior. Fight.

The MRI

Saturday, October 15, 2011

It was windy, kind of cold, with drizzly rain. Winter was coming. Bah. I much prefer warm weather. Rick ran errands; Martha was working. I wrote and wrote.

Tonight was the MRI. I couldn't eat after 4 pm, but I could drink. Water, ma'am, not booze. The MRI was going to check for any tumors the mammogram did not catch. Need I say more?

Rick took me to Henry Ford Hospital; we got there on time, got lost a little, and managed to find the MRI room in the basement. There wasn't anyone there. Rick read magazines while I watched one of the dumbest TV game shows ever produced. Then a man showed up, clearly not a receptionist, but he did the duty of one.

I was ushered back to change out of my clothes. I was the lucky recipient of my own pair of paper pants and another hospital gown, this one bigger than I needed. The technician acted surprised when I told her to stick the IV where she thought it should go; evidently not every patient was as compliant as I. Earplugs, rather unobtrusive and effective, went in next.

Yes, I had to have an IV. How else was the technician supposed to shoot the radioactive stuff into my breasts for the test? It would help the MRI locate cancer. I would drink the stuff if I had to. And yes, I had to let her shove me into the MRI tube. I forgot that I am a bit claustrophobic. I'd only had one other MRI in my whole life. That was when I discovered that I am a bit claustrophobic.

I whined, and the technician patiently pulled me out of the tube. She wanted to give me a pep talk, but all I needed to do was remind myself why I was doing this. Shove me back in and let's get this over with. I could survive half an hour or so of torture to save my life.

I was on my stomach, with my head turned to the side, my forehead on a fist so my nose didn't burrow into the towel. My breasts hung down through round holes. That was where the MRI was aiming its X-ray vision—at my breasts. Wow, no wonder they gave me earplugs. MRI machines are noisy. The first test took three minutes. I concentrated on deep breathing to control claustrophobic heebie jeebies.

During the next test, which lasted ten minutes, I discovered that claustrophobia is more manageable with the eyes open. The hospital gown and part of my arm were easier to concentrate on than blankness on the inside of my eyelids. I didn't quite understand it, though. The test was supposed to take ten minutes. It wasn't nearly that long.

The following test was the only one that couldn't be redone. The radioactive stuff got turned on and flowed through the IV into my arm. It felt cool until it passed the elbow, and then it wasn't cool anymore. I could feel it in my mouth as warmth. Then I didn't feel it at all. I was obedient and didn't move while the MRI banged away.

I did cough during the final test, which was another three minute deal, but the technician said it was okay. And I was done.

Rick and I left, me wondering where the time went. The technician told me I would be inside the tube for at least half an hour. It couldn't have been that long. It felt like ten minutes all together. But I was proud: I conquered the claustrophobia.

Please, MRI machine, do not find anything.

Monday, October 17, 2011

A computer client called, missing an important file. Tim couldn't remember the name, which told me how important the file was. I suggested it might be on one of his removable drives. If it was on the server, MozyPro should have it backed up, so all was not lost. I explained how to get files back from MozyPro.

The mailman brought a package; it was the needlepoint stocking I was going to finish for the friend of a friend.

I called to find out the results of the MRI. They were not in; the receptionist would have the nurse call me. I told her I also would like to know if my Her-2/neu was positive or negative.

My client called back. He found the lost file on one of the removable drives, just as I suggested. I am so good.

I went over what I had written, fixing errors and trying to think of amusing ways to lighten the load. Suddenly, it was 1:30 and I had not eaten. I also realized that I didn't feel stressed, I wasn't panicky. There was no lump in my gut and I could ignore that there was one in my breast. Hallelujah, a normal day.

Wednesday, October 19, 2011

Give up on normal days. Even if nothing actively happened connected with breast cancer, it dominated my life.

I was out all morning with computer work. Bill needed the capability of scanning labels into the computer and printing them out as real labels. That meant setting a scanner up on that computer, installing a graphics program, getting everything pointed to the right directory, creating a label for him to work with, and testing it. I could do it, but wondered if Bill could. He's not the most computer friendly guy. But where there is a will, there would have to be a way. If he must, Bill could call me and I'd walk him through the process over the phone.

I knew there was a reason to celebrate Alexander Graham Bell's invention, which, by the way, is said to be the most valuable patent of all time. That tidbit is courtesy of Jeopardy, the thinking person's game show. And

Bill is great—he mastered the complex task the first time he did it.

Then I treated myself to brunch at Janet's. Jerry was there; the biggest, baddest teddy bear I knew.

Jerry is one of the friendliest people in America. He meets someone and automatically becomes their friend. Generous, tolerant, God loving and the least likely to need to be God fearing, he is a friend of mine and Rick's. We are really unlikely looking friends. Dreadlocks, shoulders the width of a doorway, and black skin mean lots of people would be afraid to meet Jerry in a dark alley. Short, past pudgy into fat and gray haired, I couldn't scare a flea off a cat.

Jerry was in a bad place in the 80's. The doctors said he would be on dialysis and that was if he lived. Jerry showed them how wrong doctors can be. Now, he was having trouble with his heart and blood pressure. Undoubtedly, the heart and blood were connected, but it was a matter of the medical community connecting the dots and figuring out a fix. My big, bad teddy bear friend had an amazing attitude. He could crawl into his own problems and drown. Not Jerry.

He offered me support—he modeled the smart way of dealing with problems—he was an inspiration, but I wanted to wait a while before I went whole hog with it. Let me find out exactly how I was going to beat cancer first. Thanks to Jerry, by the time I left Janet's, I could smile.

The phone was a blessing and a curse. The doctor called. The MRI found a second dot not far from the cancer. Not to worry, the surgeon would dig it out with the first tumor. The mail came. Efficiently, Henry Ford mailed the report; I could read it myself.

The findings: nothing in the right breast, a cause for cheer, but I didn't pay much attention. I was still reading.

On the left breast, approximately 1.4 cm (centimeters) anterior to the biopsy site, there was a small 4 mm (millimeters) area of clumped enhancement/foci demonstrating slow initial enhancement with predominantly persistent kinetics. The overall extent excluding the biopsy site measured 4 cm.

I didn't like the sound of 4 cm. Was the tumor that big?

The radiologist gave his impressions so I could try to make sense of the mumbo jumbo. There was a post-biopsy change in the 5 o'clock position of the left breast, corresponding to patient's known malignancy. The 4 mm spot could represent benign tissue or DCIS. (I knew that term! DCIS meant cancer that was sitting in a milk duct, sulking because it hadn't clawed through the wall of the duct. If it was DCIS, it was the most harmless sort of tumor.) I didn't try to decipher the medicalese like 'clumped enhancement/foci'. It's a foreign language.

I was left wondering if things were worse or not. But if you consider the MRI the first hurdle to beating breast cancer, my toe got caught going over the bar. I stumbled, but didn't fall. I was still in the race for the gold.

Tomorrow was the Breast Cancer Clinic. Martha would love to go, but she had to work. Rick was going with me. Me—I was going. Had to. Didn't want to.

We made plans. Not that planning was so convoluted, but we only had one car, times were inconvenient, and I lost my efficiency somewhere. Martha had to be in Greektown at 9, Rick and I had to be at Henry Ford Hospital at 8. So Martha was going to be at work early. She didn't complain.

When I told her the results of the MRI, Martha tensed.

Damn you, Cancer. It should be a joke when they talk about being a burden to your kids.

Thursday, October 20, 2011

Dear Cancer,

I haven't even had surgery and already you are screwing up my life. Why don't you take a walk off the park pier; no one would save you from drowning in the Detroit River.

I will find a way to get rid of you. I may not sound optimistic, but I am determined. Last night, I caught myself talking about after I am rid of you. I don't have any doubt that I'll be able to banish you short term.

For most of my life I had known that five years is the magic time. If I get you out of my body, I will have to wait five years until I know if you are gone for good. If you don't come back within five years, they pronounce me cured. Mom beat the five year time bomb; she was cured of breast cancer, though effects of the treatment doomed her two decades later. Grandma's cousin beat the bomb too. As to Grandma and Mary Helen, Mom's sister, I don't know. Grandma died of another cancer and Mary Helen died before her five years were up. I just don't know. Have things changed since the 1960's? I don't think it has, not substantially.

Today is the Breast Cancer Clinic. I'll get more information—the information I need to defeat you.

I do best when I can wake naturally, usually around 8 am. If I use an alarm clock, it invariably wakes me in the middle of a dream. I am sleepy, slow, stupid for a couple of hours, until my metabolism kicks in. My metabolism has always been slow. This morning, I was up with the alarm at 6:30. I didn't feel rested; I didn't feel as if I had slept. I didn't feel ready for the day. But I was ready to leave at 7:15, as were Rick and Martha.

We were pretty quiet in the car, but it felt good to have Rick at the hospital. It's not anything I have ever said, but with Rick at my side, I am safe. No, he is not a warrior—he is a decent man who cares about me.

The clinic was less and more than I hoped for. There were five women total, all facing cancer, but we didn't introduce ourselves. We afflicted ones and supporting players watched a short video that echoed some of my Internet research and then we were ushered into individual examining rooms where we would each meet with the doctors who would save our lives.

I was the recipient of a two inch thick, well-made binder full of information, courtesy of the Josephine Ford Cancer Center. There was no time to read, but later, I would devour it.

I saw a stream of doctors, but the most valuable visit was from Barbara, the nurse coordinator. Calm, understanding, but not soppy, little nuggets of wisdom fell from her lips. Least valuable was the surgeon (not my surgeon, but the one who was supposed to give me a second opinion,) who never came to see me. Barbara thought it must be because my surgery was already scheduled, but I had questions for that man. Serious, deep questions.

God, I wanted to talk to that surgeon. The reason it mattered so much was that I had gotten one more bit of information from one of the oncologists who did come to talk to pitiful me.

I was triple negative.

No, it wasn't me that was triple negative. It was the tumor. I had triple negative breast cancer. And it was bad news.

Definition of Triple Negative Breast Cancer

What is triple negative breast cancer? It is three things:
1) The tumor is not estrogen receptive.
2) It is not progesterone receptive.
3) It is not Her-2/neu receptive.

How it got its name is obvious. Every once in a while researchers hit the nail on the head and come up with a descriptive name that doesn't need to be translated. Writing books, a name can mean the difference between good sales and a quick death. In cancer, it means the difference in what treatment is available.

Triple negative means that all the drugs that have been developed to counterattack breast cancer were useless for me. I couldn't pop a pill to kill the cancer or keep it from recurring. That's disturbing; we are conditioned from childhood that if we get sick, the doctor can give us something to help. Throw that training out the window. There weren't any pills to help me. My treatment options were limited.

Triple negative has deeper meaning. Most of the web sites on the Internet that talked about triple negative were gloomy. Triple negative tumors are more aggressive. They grow faster, spread sooner and easier, and they come back at will. They pop up here and there without warning.

The best treatment for triple negative tumors seems to be chemotherapy.

That is what the oncologists told me. When they realized I was triple negative, they changed plans for my treatment. First, I would have a lumpectomy. Because of the additional spot, they wouldn't use a melon baller on me; they were splurging on a brand new supersize ice cream scoop. Then I would have chemotherapy. I would lose my hair, no if, ands, or buts. (The upside of this is quite often the hair grows back luxuriantly.) After chemotherapy, I would have radiation, as much radiation as I could stand.

It was a more aggressive regimen, appropriate for a more aggressive malignancy.

Damn you to Hell, Cancer. It's going to be unpleasant with an ice cream scoop digging out half my breast, drugs running around my body killing harmless little cells along with yucky ones, and then a laser beam rooting around in my breast, but I'll get through it. It's the long-term I am worried about. It's harder to cure triple negative.

Change the subject so I don't cry.

Hindsight is 20/20. As soon as someone breathes the word chemotherapy in your ear, stop at the drug store and buy a good quality multivitamin and B-Complex vitamins (I ended up with Super B Complex.) Don't worry that you will overdose on Vitamin D; it won't happen, not at that dose. Start taking them now and keep taking them. The more you bolster your body, the better you will do. The B vitamins will help protect your nerves—not save them, but protect them. Neuropathy (which I discuss later) is not to laugh at.

Don't you love how I reduce the medical community to an impersonal "They?" They are individuals—one oncologist is tall for a woman and refreshingly happy to drop her professional demeanor to chat about people peeking in the hospital windows with binoculars. We were on the 13th floor (the Oncology Department is on the 13th floor of Henry Ford Hospital. I didn't think of the irony until I typed this.) Anyone determined to play Peeping Tom deserved an eyeful of me in a hospital gown.

The employees and doctors were respectful, pleasant, and obviously competent. It was the lady oncologist who discussed damage to the heart that can happen with radiation treatment. I noted she didn't promise it wouldn't happen, but she said that there had been advances in technique and equipment that help avoid that disaster.

I guess killing one killer is worth the risk of setting another killer loose. Cross your fingers that I did better than my mom. Her heart was damaged by radiation.

Encouragement came from learning that when it came to radiation, it could be done at Cottage Hospital, the same place I had my yearly mammograms. Since I would be there five days a week for six or seven weeks, the miniscule traveling distance was most convenient. If I had to, I could even take a cab without going broke. Still wouldn't shop on The Hill.

Chemotherapy would be at Henry Ford Hospital, the place we were at right now. Manageable, though a nuisance when we only had one car. Both Rick's and Martha's bosses were understanding; if one or the other had to take time off work to ferry me around, they could do it.

My last visitor at the Breast Cancer Clinic was an American Cancer Society volunteer. She loaded me down with pamphlets and cheerfully told me I was a breast cancer survivor.

Sorry, that propaganda didn't work for me. I wasn't a cancer survivor. Not yet. Not until I at least had the surgery. I told her so. She was offended, I think, but her smile didn't dim while she explained to me and Rick that I was a cancer survivor. I rejected that thinking—it didn't work for me. Yes, I'd be glad to be as optimistic as I possibly could—I would be as determined as anyone can imagine—I would fight cancer to my last breath if I had to, but I could not lie to myself and say I was a survivor. Not yet. She couldn't let it go. If I kept my mouth shut, we would have been rid of her faster, but I was compelled to argue. Finally, she was out the door.

I had to donate a bit of blood to the cause because they wanted to do a couple of tests, and then we could leave. It was past 1 pm and we were hungry.

At long last, Rick and I were outside, enjoying a semi-warm, rainy Detroit afternoon, getting our car from the valet and deciding where to eat before we keeled over. Pegasus in Greektown. They have Opa, as in flaming saganaki. Opa was worth walking a block in the rain.

Rick hadn't planned to go to work, but it was only midafternoon, and there was enough work to keep him going till doomsday. I tried to convince him that it was okay, but he intended to take me home. I mattered more than work. That's one in your eye, all you workaholic spouses.

Only once did Rick start to say something I couldn't deal with. I quickly asked him to please not be maudlin. I scarfed down my lamb and rice and then realized that Rick did the same with his gyro. We sure are a matched set.

At home, it was back to the Internet, where I learned everything reported here on triple negative. The pdf issued by Living Beyond Breast Cancer (lbbc.org) and the Triple Negative Breast Cancer Foundation was most useful. It was honest and factual. Factual equaled comforting.

For example, the pdf clearly explained, "A receptor is a protein that lives inside or on the surface of a cell and binds to something in the body to cause the cell to react." (That's how positive estrogen, progesterone and Her-2/neu feed cancer.) The pdf was as clear as it could get. I copied that file to my desktop.

Glancing at the pile of pamphlets from the American Cancer Society, I focused on the catalog. I was interested. Then I got back to life. Tomorrow I left for California. I needed to get some laundry done. Oh, Rick had started it.

Martha came home; I pushed the American Cancer Society catalog at her. "Pick out something for me," I ordered. She leafed through it and then I ordered her to give it to Rick. "Pick something out." You'd think I could do it myself, wouldn't you?

No, you don't know what was in the catalog. It was hats, turbans, scarves, and wigs. Things to cover heads gone bald by chemotherapy. Christ on a crutch, I hated things on my head. When I was little, ladies wore gloves and hats to church. Mom only made me wear a bonnet on Easter. One year. I don't remember any squabbles, but I also don't have pictures of me in hats, only the one year I wore an Easter bonnet. That was it. I hate hats.

When I got married, I flat-out refused a veil. Luella, an old friend, was scandalized that my head would be bare in church, so Mom tried flowers in my hair. She gave up. I walked down the aisle with my hair on my head and that was enough.

When it was below 0° outside, I might wear a hat—and then again, I might not. I HATE wearing things on my head.

Rick laughed when he said he couldn't imagine me wearing anything from the catalog. Martha was not far behind, but she thought I might be satisfied with a wig. I'd have to think about it. It was going to be winter when I had chemotherapy. My head was going to get cold if there wasn't any hair on it. I couldn't imagine going out in public bald; I might as well wear something. I might just turn into a hermit until something grew back.

No, I was going to wear something on my head. Christ on a crutch.

Let me diverge. What does Christ on a crutch mean? I couldn't find an answer on the Internet. I don't think it means that religion is a crutch; it sounds more like saying that we are crippling religion. Or is it just a rude way of referring to Christ on the cross?

I'd rather go into random stuff than deal with something on my head. And if I was rude to God, I'd apologize.

Friday, October 21, 2011

One couldn't get straight to Sacramento from Detroit via air. One had to go to Chicago, or Denver, or a couple of other places first. In a way, that was nice. One didn't have to sit crammed in the cattle car over six hours straight. One could walk around another airport for a while. Get something to eat, maybe have a cigarette… Look at all the pink ribbons painted on the O'Hare airport walls in honor of Breast Cancer Awareness Month.

Thanks, but no thanks. I was into temporary amnesia.

Katie was on her way back to Sacramento from Monterey; she couldn't meet me at the airport. The company receptionist volunteered to pick me up. We had fun gossiping about my daughter. They delivered me to Katie's door with a minimum of fuss and a maximum of smiles.

When I opened the door, the cats were ready to blast Katie because they had been left alone all week with just a daily visit from the cat sitter. The scolding stopped midstream; both were poleaxed at my appearance. It was enough reaction for me to get Arwen's collar on before she bolted out the door. Sibley stayed in to purr. She got a ton of pets; I had missed her also.

I was outside walking Sibley when Katie arrived. Yes, I was walking the cat. I ambled along the sidewalk; Sibley pretty much kept pace with me. We didn't go as far as previous walks; the altercation Sibley had in September with a raccoon made her cautious—fearful.

Wish I couldn't say the same for Katie. She was so glad to see me, I couldn't help thinking that she wanted to see me before I died. That was a possibility, but no way. I was so not doing that. Sometime in the next two weeks, we would have to hash it out, but Katie was exhausted. We cuddled and went to bed when I couldn't keep my eyes open. It was 9:30 pm Sacramento time.

Sunday, October 23, 2011

Katie was vegetating, watching NCIS LA episodes, so I took myself off to see Lynda, my friend in Sacramento. Lynda is an old neighbor of Katie's, wheelchair-bound with more physical problems than I wished to face.

We talked recipes, since Lynda had rallied sufficiently to cook. The next time I came, I would bring recipes and trade. I also poured it out, all the nasty details. Lynda offered a hug, but I told her it was okay. Hugs hurt her and I could get by.

But talking to my friend coalesced my feelings. I didn't fear the surgery; it would be painful, and I was not into pain, but I would survive it. Chemotherapy bothered me; while I was not vain, I didn't like the idea of losing my hair. Radiation would be an irritation of my spirit as well as of my skin, which I understood was the worst side effect. No, what bothered me was that I had an intimation of mortality.

It was when I thought of the future that I choked up. I could die. Cancer could beat every effort and rot my insides until I died. This feeling was buried deep; it didn't surface often, but it was there. Don't deny its existence, but find a way to deal with it. I was not going to spend the next six months, not to mention the next five years, fighting tears every time I thought of the future.

Tuesday, October 25, 2011

I mulled it over and decided to email Dr. Chirurgus my questions. If I called, he would want to call back, and I was in California, for Pete's sake. I'd find out how computer savvy he was. I had two questions.
- Was my tumor the basal type?
- Was it fast growing?

Both questions related to triple negative. Basal means the cells of the tumor look like the cells that line breast ducts (where the milk flows when you breastfeed a baby.) Basal-like cancer tends to be more aggressive. This aggressiveness is not the aggressiveness of triple negative cancers—it gets its own rating. So, if I had aggressive triple negative combined with aggressive basal-like, things got scarier.

Then I pulled out all the paper I got at the Breast Cancer Clinic and started reading. The pamphlets from the American Cancer Society were repetitive; I could throw half of them away. A few would be useful—one had exercises for after surgery, another discussed Lymphedema, a chronic condition that can occur after having lymph nodes removed. I'd hang on to them. The two thickest pamphlets, For Women Facing Breast Cancer and the Breast Cancer Dictionary, might come in handy.

I would show the tlc catalog to Katie if she wasn't too tired to look. I wanted a laugh.

Last was the black binder from the Breast Cancer Clinic. I was going to read it straight through, and hadn't had time. Hadn't taken the time. Well, now I would.

This was a source of solid, unadulterated data. How to prepare for a lumpectomy; what to expect afterwards. Descriptions of blood tests, x-ray type exams, temporary conditions caused by treatments both chemo and radiation, diets—that black binder was full of information. It sure wasn't a fairy tale. The overall impression was grim.

Surgery is the least of what happens. Chemotherapy poisons the body, so much so that one has to be careful that the excretions of the body—certainly not confined to vomit—are handled carefully so as not to harm the handler. Translation: if I threw up on the bed sheets, don't touch it. Bundle the bedding up and wash it separately from everything else. Clean up any spatters with paper towels and make sure the garbage bag is sealed tightly. Rubber gloves were advisable.

Radiation treatment wasn't much better. I might not be a leper, but my vomit would be. For God's sake, don't ask to drink out of my glass.

I could run through a laundry list of the side effects I might suffer, but it was too depressing. Fatigue, hair loss, and problems with food in every way imaginable were enough for now. I can't say I was ever a health nut, but I cringed at how the doctors were going to poison me to poison my enemy.

Wednesday, October 26, 2011

Dear Cancer,
You aren't winning the mind game. I am sleeping well; no bad dreams, no insomnia. In fact, I was up early to take Katie to meet her ride, and I got to watch the sun come up over Sacramento County. The road was long and straight, going from Citrus Heights towards Highway 99, passing isolated subdivisions once it got away from "town." There weren't many trees to block the horizon, so I got to see a swatch of pretty orange red gold from side to side. I didn't actually see the sun burst over the colors, but who can beat God's skill in watercoloring the sky?

I spent the morning going through recipes with Lynda. She had a few I was interested in, especially pudding cookies. How can you go wrong putting chocolate pudding into cookie dough? I was going to email her a bunch to print out. Lynda was most interested in ways to shove disguised vegetables at her son; I wanted yummy.

Katie was gone on an audit. Yes, it was quiet, but I was comfortable with quiet. All those years of Rick traveling for work while the girls were in school taught me to enjoy solitude. You can hear the clock. Maybe some people don't like the sound, but it doesn't bother me.

The email to the doctor did not go through; he wasn't computer savvy. I would call and find out how fast the cancer was growing and how much I should fear it. Today I could stick my tongue out at it.

Nah nah nah nah nahhh nah.

Saturday, October 29, 2011

What a nice day. I hardly thought about cancer. Katie and I went shopping at the Galleria, the exclusive shopping mall for Sacramento. There, we browsed the most plebian store in the acres of stores: Sears.

Sears had the largest selection of plus-size women's nightgowns and robes and I wanted button in front whatever for the great siege. The store, basic as much of its merchandise is, had the nightgown I loved so well it grew holes—I grabbed one in my size. It wasn't button down but pullover, but I should be able to wear a regular nightgown eventually. I also got a housecoat, an honest to god old lady housecoat that snapped down the front. Katie said it was ugly, but it wasn't so bad. The print was white and cherry. I liked cherry. Cheery. And when I didn't need it any more, I wouldn't miss it.

At the register, I found out that nightgown and housecoat were both on sale. My bank account appreciated cheap nightwear. Just wait until the medical bills started rolling in. I wouldn't be able to afford lint.

We stopped at Katie's office to pick up some papers. Her co-worker Mike was there, no one else, so we were in and out quickly. The drug store had Katie's allergy medicine; the poor girl was sneezing up a storm. I told her five years ago that she should continue her allergy shots, but when was she to fit the doctor's visits into her schedule? No one listens to a mother's wisdom (fine, call it nagging.)

It was warm enough that I left my sweater in the car. Got to love California—at least when it is in the 30's in Detroit. Martha had to scrape the windows of the car. Maybe I'd stay in Sac... No, I just wished I could.

Back home, Katie held a conversation with Arwen. The cat, Arwen, who spent the week avoiding me. Her collar had been on day and night since she wouldn't let me near her to take it off. I fed the cat, opened doors in the morning so she could go out and closed them at night so she was safe inside. Her litter box was clean and a few toys were tossed around. Only a few—Arwen had been avoiding me. Katie said, "You shouldn't avoid Mom, Arwen. She's nice."

We talked about the trick or treating thing at the church. We were supposed to be in costume, but the theme was Wild West. There wasn't a thing we could do to fit that theme. I offered to dress all in black and be the Wicked Witch of Detroit, but Katie said, "No, no one will believe it. You're too nice."

I got fuzzy warm feelings. How wonderful is it to have your daughter think you are nice?

Martha went shopping. She got some clothes, which she sorely needed, and found a red hat for me. It was soft and stretchy, just what she thought would suit me when I went bald. I hoped it matched the cherry housecoat and got more fuzzy warm feelings that she was thinking of me.

Rick painted the window on the stairs. Bless him. He also talked to Joann, who went through the breast cancer rigmarole a couple of years ago. Joann wanted me to call; knowing her, she would be honest and I would be better prepared for what came. I wished Rick didn't sound so down.

I didn't spend the day immersed in cancer. It felt good.

Tuesday, November 1, 2011

My emotions were on a rollercoaster. Or as a character emphasized in a Jane Austen movie, "I can't get out. I can't get out."

Sunday night was plain old fun. Katie and I handed out Halloween candy to enough children to populate a town—which they do. Katie's church, one of those mega-churches, hosts the area's young the night before Halloween with a fair. There was a Ferris wheel, at least five bounce houses, police cars and fire trucks to climb on, a huge slide, a climbing wall, and a line of cars in the parking lot equipped with candy and willing folks to hand it out. We were but one car of at least thirty. I smiled so much my face felt split, but it was a happy smile.

Katie did most of the work. I didn't have any stamina.

Yesterday rolled around. The doctor's office called promptly at 9 am. They were obviously wise to the time difference between Detroit and Sacramento. They could have called at 6.

They didn't know if the malignancy was basal or not, nor did they know how quickly it was growing. But Dr. Chirurgus had had a death in the family; he would like to attend the funeral and be with the family.

Could we postpone the surgery a week?

Ooh, a rock dropped into my stomach. Delay the operation? Was it safe to do so? Would the cancer grow like a weed and spread to my lymph nodes? Spread throughout my body and choke me to death? Dr. Chirurgus' opinion was it should make no difference to wait a week. I weakly agreed to postpone the surgery.

Then I called Rick. He was at work, swamped and sounding defeated. The next call was to the American Cancer Society to ask their opinion. Their phone system was simple to get through, but talking to a person didn't happen. The phone rang and rang and no one answered. It was a conspiracy. No, there was no conspiracy. With the logical kernel of my brain I knew all the people were busy. I waited a few minutes and called back.

I already knew what the woman told me, so she found a medical person to talk to me. I had difficulty articulating my concern to the next person. A few frustrating minutes later, she gave me a clue. I should talk to members of the team in charge of my care; they were the ones who could advise me.

Rick called Joe's wife, who was an oncology nurse for Henry Ford Health System downriver. She said a week was not going to make any difference. That calmed me. I was glad I got a sensible answer from her.

So why was I weepy?

Thursday, November 3, 2011

I found a dimple on my breast over the biopsy site. It gave me a scare, and then logic told me it was related to the biopsy. Deciding I would have to call Dr. Chirurgus' office, I went to bed. For the first time, I found it difficult to sleep.

The surgeon must be psychic; his nurse, Connie, called at 6:15 am. She forgot the time difference, but I didn't mind. It was better to get everything squared away. It was Connie's opinion that the dimple meant nothing, but I should watch for signs of infection and call immediately if the area looked worse. She asked how I was doing and I was honest, telling her of my unease with the postponement of the surgery. She said she would see if she could move the date up.

I was up; the cats were glad to be fed. They went back to sleep and I turned on my laptop to check my email. Connie called back; the surgery would be Wednesday, November 16, instead of Friday the 18th. Ridiculous to feel relief over a few measly days, but I felt better. Maybe it was more that I wished to be in control. Who cares?

As I wrote, I couldn't deny that my breast was a bit tender. I looked in the mirror and didn't notice any difference. I hoped it didn't mean anything, but I would keep track of the dimple.

Monday, November 7, 2011

Dear Cancer,
Home again, home again, jiggedy jig. Yes, I was home from Sacramento. Usually, I spent the last few days at Katie's wanting to be both there and at home, and then, when I got home, I wanted to be back at Katie's. Rick understands this awful feeling of wanting to be two places at once; I think that is why he never complained about me spending so much time in California.

This time, I didn't want to come home. Now that I was home, I wanted only to be in Sacramento. This didn't have anything to do with family or cats. Nothing personal, but I had this irrational feeling that if I stayed in Sac, you, Cancer, could be ignored. The mind is a wondrous thing. Thank God I am more sensible than my irrational thoughts.

I finally saw Dr. Sanatio, fearless doctor and friend. My excuse was that my right ear was sensitive to sound on the plane, which meant my sinuses were infected again. They get boggy, then it goes in my ears, and then it is time for antibiotic. It's a chronic problem.

Going to see him was not stressful. How could I claim that when I was facing a possible death sentence? Maybe because my blood pressure was 117 over 72. Seeing Dr. Sanatio was helpful, not stressful. He wouldn't lie to me—he wouldn't hide anything—he would be truthful.

He was. Dr. Sanatio told me that I was having a surgical procedure, nothing more. A lumpectomy was not a big deal. No six inch scars, no weeks of horrendous pain. Stop agonizing over it. Until we knew if the lymph nodes were affected or pathology came up with more, I should leave it at that. I respond well to matter-of-fact. Thank you, Dr. Sanatio.

I told him about the American Cancer Society volunteer and her, "You are a cancer survivor," and he understood why I felt she was silly, but he wanted me to keep the attitude, if not the words. Be optimistic. I would do better overall if I could do that.

I felt more optimistic. A chip had fallen off my shoulder.

Wednesday, November 9, 2011

A lady called from the hospital doing a pre-surgery questionnaire. She asked a ton of questions. Had I ever had surgery before? Any allergies?

What medications did I take? The only order I got was to not take Naproxen, the pills I popped when my back started to stiffen up.

When my back goes, I get migraine-like headaches. She suggested Tylenol as a substitute for Naproxen, as if that would be any help if I wanted to bang my head against the wall for relief from pain. Behave, back. Other body parts took precedence.

Friday, November 11, 2011

Oh frabjous day, callooh callay! (that's how Lewis Carroll spelled it.) Today was 11-11-11. Something like that doesn't roll around every day. The last time we got a date that really stuck in my mind was 7-7-77; my nephew was born the day before. It was cold and still damp, but we were going out for dinner to celebrate. That was my executive decision, and it was final. Not that Rick would have a problem with it.

I was into indulging myself. I like going out to dinner. I was spending money on my genealogy. I ordered a marriage record through ancestry.com for the brother of my 3 times great-grandfather, looking for clues to their father's death date. I authorized a genealogy service to spend $150 looking for Joseph Keeler and his father in Ohio. 4 times great-grandfather Joseph is what they call a brick wall; I can't find him. I know his name and that is all.

I bought a $20 lottery ticket that could turn me into a millionaire. Better late than never! Stop the negativity, Ann. It is never late when you are talking about honey-falls.

Individually, I could afford to do the things I mentioned, but I tried to limit the doing especially for genealogy, which can be an expensive habit. We were not rich, after all. But now, I felt unfettered from our budget; I wanted to indulge myself. It was the fault of the malignancy in my breast.

I never before felt that life was too short to do everything, but now I understood the urgency. Life can be too short. It wasn't going to be too short for me (see, Dr. Sanatio, I did feel optimistic) but I didn't want to waste time.

See how a serious illness changes your thinking?

The other activity I undertook was something beyond my understanding. I was cooking casseroles and freezing them. It is one of the chores I do for Katie, but why do it for Rick, Martha and myself? It is not usual behavior. I enjoy doing genealogy much more than I enjoy cooking. The last time I had surgery, when they straightened the septum of my nose, I knew ahead of time that I would be off in La La Land for a good week and

I didn't do any extra cooking. I didn't cook up a storm before I left Detroit to go to Sacramento. I was not going to worry about it, but I did have plans to cook two more meals. One would be eaten tomorrow (remember my decision to go out to dinner) and the second would be frozen.

My self-indulgence would have to take a break. I had to sew a needlepoint Christmas stocking.

Saturday, November 12, 2011

The best laid plans of mice and men aft gang aglay (or however Bobby Burns spelled it.) No going out to dinner last night; Rick didn't get home until 8:30. Martha and I were starved, so we ordered pizza. Almost as good as going out, right?

The stocking was half sewn. Rick and I ran errands together; he had to get stuff for the snow blower and I needed fresh pineapple (one of my favorite snacks) and something to attach to that Christmas stocking as a hanger.

Rick and I talked in the car. He was stressed—work, money, and me. Work has been a pain for years, chill out. Money—let's worry about that later. Me, well, just love me and think good thoughts. We cleared the air.

When we got home, the mailman had delivered the first of an endless string of bills from Henry Ford. $863.00 due by the end of the month. What a laugh. I'd call them Monday and tell them what we could afford monthly. Or should I wait until after the lumpectomy? No, Henry Ford was pretty reasonable.

Surgery

Suggested Shopping List

- Loose shirt to wear to the hospital and a loose nightgown or pajamas—all buttoning/snapping in front. The hospital may ask that you bring a robe; you may not be able to lift your arms to pull on shirts and nightgowns.
- Pain medication that will be prescribed by the surgeon (ask for the script ahead of time)
- A couple of drinking straws (optional)
- Extra pillows so you don't lay flat in bed (optional)
- Sponge bath supplies (I used Oil of Olay wipes) (optional)

Tuesday, November 15, 2011

It was the day before Doomsday. I hadn't taken a shower yet; I was working on another computer. Doesn't it figure that just before I went hors de combat, everyone wanted my services. One sad sack laptop, a printer to install, a new client to train, a needlepoint pillow to block and sew. Rick would pick up the slack on the computer work. Didn't need to lose clients.

Lumpectomies filled my thoughts. It started Sunday night, this obsession with the surgery. The little knot of dread floated in and out of my stomach.

I'd talked to a couple of people who'd had lumpectomies and they assured me it wasn't bad, but I had trouble believing them. It was a combination of the amount the surgeon was going to dig out with the ice cream scoop combined with the need for the edges of the melon to be cancer free, along with the determination that my lymph nodes had to be spotless, that made me nervous.

The lumpectomy's location made a difference in how it felt.

A bout with cancer is an obstacle course. One has to clear all the obstacles to win. I semi-failed the first hurdle—the MRI. Rather than coming up with only the expected, the MRI found a bit more. The surgery was the second and third hurdles. A clear, clean margin (edge) around what they removed would mean the better the chances they got the entire tumor. I requested a remarkably wide, clear as day margin. No involvement of lymph nodes; pray that my malignancy was retarded and couldn't figure out how to get to lymph nodes.

I was glad I opted to have surgery on Wednesday rather than Friday. Enough waiting. It was time to get moving on this. It felt a little like waiting for Christmas—hurry up and happen. It just wasn't a good feeling.

Thanksgiving was the following week; the question would be could I drive to Lansing to celebrate with the family? Could my poor abused breast tolerate being jounced around in a car for four hours? Who knows? I was uncomfortable after the biopsy; I could feel the bouncy bouncy of my breast. Michigan's roads are not smooth so there would be lots of bouncy bouncy. Rick would like to go; he doesn't see his family often. I urged him to wait and see. Carol could deal with three people more or less eating her turkey and green bean casserole.

Rick decided to stay home. That was good. The doctor said to stay home.

My back behaved; the Naproxen sat in its bottle, ignored. I finished sewing the Christmas stocking. Had to pack and ship it.

The billing department at Henry Ford Health System wasn't busy; I got a guy on the phone right away. He set up a payment plan of $100 per month without question. I'd up the amount after the first of the year when one of our big payments was done. Doesn't it figure—pay off something big and something else takes its place.

You should see everything that needed doing around the house. Dust, blow away.

Wednesday, November 16, 2011

Lumpectomy Day. Should be a national holiday, don't you think?

One could tell today was special by the way I woke up. The alarm rang at 7 and I jolted up. For someone who usually lolls in bed nudging her metabolism to get a move on, I did pretty well. If it hadn't been forbidden, I would have taken Naproxen; my back was stiffening up and I had a slight headache from it. It was that time of year. Cold and dampness upsets the abused muscles in my back. Oh well, I'd be so medicated, I wouldn't notice.

Rick headed for the shower and I spent fifteen minutes reading a book, then I got dressed in the button up the front shirt, as ordered, and sweats.

The few things I needed to take to Macomb Hospital were in a pile in front of the computer, ready to go. Some paperwork, my driver's license and Blue Cross card, directions to the hospital—that's all I needed. Everything else was connected to my feet.

Martha bummed a ride to work from a co-worker, so we didn't have to deliver her to the office in Greektown.

Rick and I were going in the opposite direction, away from rush hour. As a result, we got to the general location of Macomb Hospital and had plenty of time to get confused. Considering the hospital was nearly an hour away, up by the "new" mall, we were doing pretty well. But Henry Ford Health System needed to put up a few more directional signs. A road that circles the complex in one fell swoop would be a bonus. There was one, but it didn't go all the way around. At least I didn't think it did. We missed the road we were supposed to turn on and Rick had to make a U-turn to get into the correct parking lot.

He delivered me to the covered portico and then went to park the car. I made a mental note to remember how to get there; I wasn't sure if I would have to come back.

Inside, the first door to my left was the Operative Center, where I was to sign in. I gave my name at the desk and Rick and I sat to watch TV. Whatever show was on, they were interviewing the winners (or finalists) of Dancing for the Stars. I never watched Dancing for the Stars and had no interest in the stars, the steps or missteps and gossip; I people watched. It must have been Old People Day. Everyone in the waiting room was a good 20-30 years older than I.

I was called to the desk to sign in. A woman with a lovely contralto voice asked questions, chief of which were, "Why are you here?" and "Which breast," did the paperwork, and told us that they were short on beepers; Rick would get one later.

Then I was ushered to the Pre-Op area, which was also the Post-Op area. I was assigned Bed 25 and a very nice nurse named Sue, who asked "Why are you here" and "Which breast," then gave me a big hospital gown, tacky slipper socks, and a bag to put my clothes in, and joy of joys, an IV port and two somethings that I couldn't see slapped on the underside of my breast to numb it. I think they were patches, but as I said, I couldn't see them, and I was not into asking questions.

Once I looked like an honest to God patient, Sue gave me a Valium. It was welcome; I was breathing faster than normal and feeling weepy. By the time she allowed Rick in, I was mildly loopy—certainly happier than I was before popping the pill. My breathing evened out and I could joke, but I didn't like finding out that I would have a breathing tube during surgery. That made it sound like hard core surgery. Thank God for Valium. I could keep my cool.

Rick and I had a few minutes together. He wanted to hold my hand and be supportive. I wanted him to talk about anything other than medical anything.

At 9:30, I was bundled into a wheelchair to go for the Wire Localization—translated into English, to have guide wires stuck in my tumor so the surgeon could find the malignancy without trouble. The surgery was at 1 pm; I was going to have wires sticking out of my breast all morning? Sounded nasty, but I didn't question it.

Wheeling around under the power of a twenty-something girl, I suggested running over any people who looked like surgeons. She was cheerful, but failed to bump into anyone.

Cheerful girl and I had to go way to the other end of the hospital complex. It was a long hike through corridors, past the main lobby and gift shop, through more corridors. Other than wishing to bowl them over, I was not fazed by people along the way. Valium freed me from normal inhibitions. Evidently, hospital gowns and weird slipper socks are fashionable enough, because I didn't notice anyone staring.

I felt sorry for my chair pusher having to haul my excessive weight around, but she wasn't even breathing hard. She must be used to fat ladies.

Arriving at the proper place, the name of which escaped me, I found I was second in line. The woman in the wheelchair in front of me was asleep. I was offered a magazine; I flipped through it but had trouble focusing. Whoops, Valium did more than relax. It made me sleepy. As in really sleepy. When I was not dozing, I realized I was in the mammography department for the Wire Localization procedure. A couple of women arrived, I think for mammograms; one looked apprehensive, the other bored. I didn't notice when they left. I vaguely registered the departure of the woman ahead of me in the wheelchair line.

The room must be right off the corridor, but for the life of me, I couldn't remember how I got there. My trusty wheelchair was gone; I was operating under my own power. It was my turn with my old friend, the mammogram machine, except it didn't look like the machine at Cottage Hospital's Woman's Center. Oh, it was a digital one.

I got to sit on a chair, but it came out of Quasimodo's laboratory. It was a deformed secretarial rolling chair: short seat, short back tilted forward, and a bit high off the ground so I was on tiptoe, not flatfooted. Even for befuddled-on-Valium patients, it was not comfortable. Technicians floated around, coming and going.

My hospital gown had snaps on the left sleeve so I didn't have to remove it for my breast to go into the machine. The technicians were impressed that my snaps snapped and unsnapped without a fight. Amazing the details that matter. I'd like to take credit for working snaps, but I kept my mouth shut except to answer the question, "Which breast?" I was too high to do more than obey instructions.

My friend Sue (from church) told me about her experience with Wire Localization. She had to stand and a technician was on the floor in front of her, looking up. She didn't tell me that my breast was not squished nearly as flat as when a mammogram is the object. Overall, Sue had the economy experience and I the deluxe procedure: I got a weird chair and two technicians stooping at my left side.

The Wire Localization was done much as the biopsy was accomplished. A big needle was inserted into my breast and the wire went in via the needle. The patches Nurse Sue glued to my breast were useful; I didn't feel a thing.

The first wire was a breeze, but the second was at an awkward angle. They made an adjustment or two, and then I was wheeled out with tape covering my wires.

Doped, I hoped the surgeon could get the wires out. I'd hate to walk around the rest of my life with two wires in my breast. I couldn't feel them with my left arm, so they must not have stuck out very far, but I could still feel them. No, that's not the Valium talking. I could feel that there was something at the left edge of my breast where it faded into my chest, but I couldn't feel anything with my arm, which brushed against the area. It was the Valium's fault that I irrationally focused on something that was but wasn't there.

My next appointment was in Nuclear Medicine for the Sentinel Node Indicator procedure. I didn't recall getting there, but it wasn't the same place as the Mammography department. The walls were dingier than in the "public" areas of the hospital. Or was it just less lit? Or was I so stoned on Valium?

I lay on the table that slid into a donut x-ray machine. It reminded me of the MRI machine, but a lot more open. The girl running it asked, "Which breast?" and shot ink and radioactive junk into my breast. Then the donut slid over me rather than me sliding into it. I was staring at a white plate divided into four sections. It hovered over me, but was nothing overwhelming to claustrophobic folks.

We took a picture for five minutes, waited five or ten minutes and took another five minute picture, looking to see where the ink went. Sometimes it takes half an hour for the ink to get moving, I was assured, but I didn't have a cooperative breast. I lost track of how many pictures were taken; three, four, five? But the ink didn't move much.

It would be up to Dr. Chirurgus to figure out in surgery where the ink traveled and which lymph node(s) to remove. Time flies when you are having fun; I didn't have a clue how long I lay on the table, but it certainly wasn't as long as ten minutes.

After I said goodbye to the donut, Sue huffed up to wheel me back to Pre-Op. I'd been gone a long time; the doctor was looking for me. Tick up another side effect of Valium. I couldn't care less that the surgeon was looking for me. I'm not sure I understood what he wanted with me.

Back at Bed 25, the clock said 12:30. I lost an hour or so, didn't I? While I marveled at the time, things happened, the most important of them being Dr. Chirurgus arrived.

While the surgeon asked "Which breast?" and marked my shoulder with a checkmark marks the spot, Sue put my IV together and shot medicine in. It was uncomfortably cold and she assured me it would be over soon. She was right; I didn't remember anything else until I woke up in Bed 25.

I was dreaming; I had to match everything up. They were in squares, maybe people? People sitting in dark 3-D squares? Still, I had to match them up. I was close to completion, but Sue and Rick interrupted. I managed to link up two more squares, and then decided it was time to fight myself awake. The times I have had anesthesia, I sailed through. No drowsing for hours, no problems. I maintained my record and cleared my head.

Sometime while I was doing the matchy matchy thing, Rick talked to Dr. Chirurgus, who was quite satisfied with the surgery. He removed two lymph nodes.

Telling me that I was a cheap date, Sue untaped and slid the IV port out of my wrist. What? Oh, yes, the Valium and the sedative in the IV. I'm that way with booze also; it doesn't take much to get me loopy.

Rick helped me dress. I was glad I wore sweat pants; they went on fairly easily once Rick got them past the socks. I didn't even consider wearing the bra, which tells you I was still high. Rick pulled the shirt up my arms and buttoned me. Then my sweater went over the shirt and I was ready to leave.

He went to bring the car to the door and Sue wheeled me out in a wheelchair. In the car I became aware that I was numb to the gills; the ride was not painful. I seemed to have a bra on the left side; no, it was bandages of some sort.

My mouth and throat felt dry as dust, so we stopped at a McDonald's for a Coke. It was nearly 6 pm; we ran by the pharmacy to get the pain prescription filled (Tylenol 3 with codeine—no wimpy stuff.) Rick ran in, I waited in the car. Then he was helping me up the front steps of the house. Home again, home again, jiggedy jig.

First things first; I had to change because I wet the sweats. Not much, and no one laughed or winced. I pulled on pajama bottoms and left the shirt and sweater alone. Then I was in the living room in the comfy chair to finally, finally, FINALLY, relax. Recover. Take inventory and make sure I was still alive.

I watched Ghosthunters, ignored the phone, and dozed. The pain pills were a godsend; I was most definitely not into pain. I was supposed to use my arm, but not lift it more than 90°. No problem. I was proud that my arm worked and I used it pain free. It was more comfortable if my arm was away from my side—I propped it on the arm of the chair.

My feet weren't as cooperative; I shuffled to the bathroom. Dopey or not, I noticed that my urine was a lovely shade of blue. That was the dye from the lymph node test escaping. My throat was sore from the breathing tube; chicken soup hurt. I was too sleepy to think.

Did I watch Ghost Hunters?

Drinking through a straw was preferable to tilting a glass. Don't know why it was so, but the McDonald's straw got rinsed out and put in my water glass. Martha ran to the store for straws. (How many times can I mention how wonderful my kids are? Martha is my littlest angel, though she is now taller than I.)

Food went in my mouth at regular intervals. If I thought about it, I would have to say I was "grazing" rather than eating meals. There was no upset stomach.

I spent the entire night in the chair, with my feet up on the footstool, an afghan covering my legs, anchored by two cats who managed to squeeze together between my knees without fighting.

Friday, November 18, 2011

Yesterday was much like Wednesday night. I slept, dozed when I didn't sleep, took pain pills on schedule, ate and slept again. Rick stayed home to tend me and ended up working on a laptop and a desktop for clients.

Nurses called to check on me twice. My foggy memory thinks the first was surgical Sue and the second was Connie, Dr. Chirurgus' office nurse. She set up the follow-up visit for next Wednesday. The only other call I took was from Katie. I wanted her to know I was alive, but I wasn't chatty. Not witty. Not all there.

I had a persistent itch on my back, kind of under my left arm. I pulled my shirt up (carefully, since I was not as graceful as I could be) and Martha located the itch and scratched over the tape covering it. She couldn't see what caused the itch, but it tormented me most of the night.

I thought about sleeping prone in bed; tried it and it didn't feel good, so I spent another night in the chair. Don't cry for me, Argentina, I sleep in that chair quite often. It's comfortable, just the right angle to support my head and easy to sleep in. This time, my back got a little sore. I'm not sure if it is that I was not holding my torso normally or if it is just my back doing its thing. Still, I stayed away from the Naproxen; it wouldn't get along with the pain pills.

This morning when I woke was the first time that the Tylenol 3's were not at full dosage. Wow. The pain was not unbearable, but it was unpleasant. I was not about to wean myself from pain pills. With the drug in my system, I was comfortable. So comfortable, I could type this.

My breast was wearing a bandage. It looked like a clumsy version of what the Viking lady wears in the opera —the round pointed metal plate—except I only had the one.

Poor boobie was smaller than the right side now. That I could tell. Nothing else looked disturbed. I couldn't see any bruises. I could still feel where the two wires were; the bandage was lumpy against my arm.

The tape around the edge of the bandage ran under my arm, skimming the armpit, with tape high on my chest keeping everything up. What it looked like on the underside of my breast was unknown. I was not up to inspecting myself in a mirror.

I did have a couple of scrapes inside my mouth thanks to the breathing tube, but they were not serious or terribly painful. Everything else was in working order.

Well, almost everything. I was constipated, but didn't feel constipated. No bowel movement since Tuesday equals constipation, right? I raided Martha's store of Fiber One bars for bulk.

Martha was working from home so she could take care of me. Rick had a bad congestive cough but went to work. I arranged for Martha to ferry him to the doctor. We did NOT need Rick sick.

I could not take a bath or a shower—how to keep clean was something to worry about later. I was supposed to do sponge baths, but how? I didn't feel really dirty. My hair was starting to look bad, but I could go another day until it got frightful. Washing hair stumped me. Maybe I should go to a hairdresser to have it done. Cleanliness might be next to godliness, but I was barely awake. I couldn't quite wrap my brain around a plan. The anesthetic was out of my system, I would guess, but I still planned a serious nap for the afternoon. Tomorrow I would work on clean.

For the lady from the American Cancer Society, today was the first day I would consider being a cancer survivor.

Monday, November 21, 2011

Hey, Cancer, I know how you hang on my every word. Sorry I missed a few days; have to catch up. It won't take long.

Rick had bronchitis. There were antibiotics to take and a variety of over-the-counter products to help his cough. I apologized for not noticing him being sick. Yes, he is a full grown man and could take himself to the doctor, but he is a full grown man and failed to take himself to the doctor. That is part of my job—it says so on the marriage certificate in invisible ink.

Yesterday, I couldn't stand my head anymore. My scalp was crawling and every time I scratched it, my fingernails turned black. So Rick washed my hair in the kitchen sink, using the sprayer. We draped a towel over my left shoulder to make sure the bandage didn't get wet. Ignore that my right sleeve got soaked. The saints be praised, my hair was clean.

Not so my body. I was supposed to do sponge baths. What a laugh. Last night I had Rick run an Oil of Olay face wipe over my back and in my armpits, which were starting to stick together. Don't tell me to use a wash cloth; Rick was not the most competent nurse. I was afraid that a wet washcloth would be too bulky to get under my left armpit without wetting the bandage. My instructions were to not get the bandage wet; if I did, I had to go in and have it changed. The Olay wipe worked pretty darn well.

I wiped my chest, neck, stomach, and other needy body parts, removing a skin colored powder from my chest. I wasn't sure what it was—it went up to my chin.

I could do without the Tylenol 3, but took it on an extended schedule. I couldn't think of any reason to put up with discomfort and the pills made it go away. What did I mean by discomfort? At this point, itchiness was the main problem. I itched from the tape of the bandage. Every once in a while, I got a twinge from the underside or the far left side of my breast. Whether it was from incisions, shifting of my innards, or the tape, I couldn't tell.

When I walked, I was too aware of bouncy bouncy breast. When I used my left arm, it rubbed against my breast and made it ache. Tylenol whisked those irritations under the rug and I was not too proud to use the crutch, though I could live without it.

But there wasn't a lot of pain involved with the lumpectomy. My arm was operational, I could now sleep in bed using two or three pillows, and my appetite was normal. The constipation resolved itself after I ate a full dinner Saturday night. I was pretty much back to normal.

They treat breast cancer differently than in the past. The past I remember was the summer of 1968. My family had packed me off for a vacation with a friend. The plan was for my family to drive to Lansing to pick me up and visit my grandmother. Boy, was I surprised when I was told my uncle was flying to Lansing in his plane to pick me up.

It was the first time I flew in an airplane. That flight was loads of fun for my twelve-year-old self. I had my father and my uncle to myself in a little Cherokee and a nice long ride looking down on Michigan. When we landed at Detroit City Airport, my aunt asked, "Have you told her yet?" That was how I found out my mother was in the hospital with breast cancer. It's curious that 50 years later, I can hear my aunt asking that question. I think my world stopped for a moment. (Lesson learned: ask someone to watch over the kids during this difficult time. They need TLC and you aren't in a position to provide it.)

I don't have detailed memories of the rest of that summer. I was expected to keep house; my two older brothers maintained the outside, an equitable arrangement to a flaming male chauvinist like my father. When I got home from my vacation, Mom had been in the hospital a week; every pair of shoes my father and brothers owned was in the living room. One brother had tried to do laundry and walked the washing machine until it unplugged itself from the electrical socket.

We had a mangle—a long round iron like dry cleaners used. I had to feed the sheets through it—two passes per sheet, after I washed and dried them, and then make the beds. I probably wasn't smartass enough to say, "Dirty sheets are good for the soul." (Remembering those sheets, I fail to understand why the sheets you buy today are not wrinkle-free.)

I cooked all the meals, except the night my brothers went fishing. I flat out refused to clean the fish. I think we ordered pizza. But I discovered that I made City Chicken better than my mother; my friend's mother told me how to make gravy.

Mom was in the hospital for weeks. I do not recall seeing her; I don't believe I talked to her on the phone. The night she came home, she cooked dinner. I found out later she wasn't supposed to do any lifting, but she took over the house immediately. I was so relieved; I thought I was going to have a breakdown from the workload. Remember, I was twelve.

Maybe that is where my weak sense of "Cleanliness is next to Godliness" comes from. I think a little dirt is good for the soul. (My daughter's allergist agrees. He says that if I hadn't exposed baby Katie to a little dirt, her allergies would be more serious.)

Mom had a dressing on her chest. She changed it, but I never saw her do it. I have no idea how long it took her to heal; I did not know what had been done to her, except that the doctor had cut off her breast.

I learned later that the cancer went into her lymph nodes so the surgeon dug out all the lymph nodes on that side. The dressing on her chest got smaller, but she had it on forever because during radiation they burned a hole in her chest that never healed. I understood that you could see her rib through the hole, but she never showed it to me.

She must not have had chemo; she never lost her hair and she never told me she had it. In retrospect, the many weeks Mom spent in the hospital began with surgery for a radical mastectomy along with a full hysterectomy, followed by however much radiation. She did it without support because the boys were boys, I was too young to really help, her family was in Lansing, and my father was repelled by her disfigurement.

After that hellish summer, I knew that if she made it five years without the cancer coming back, she would be cured. More than fifteen years later, she was being tested at the same hospital where I had just given birth to Katie. Mom was exuberant when she told me there was no cancer found and then we went to the nursery to admire my baby.

Medical treatment is really different now, isn't it? And my husband is nothing like my father.

I have not agonized over you, Mr. Cancer, not since I actively began fighting your influence. Don't try to do to me what you did to Mom. I won't let you.

Wednesday Rick goes with me to Dr. Chirurgus' office to see what Pathology says. That is my hurdle. Clean lymph nodes and wide clear margins, please, God.

Tuesday, November 22, 2011

Out of curiosity, I looked up mastectomies. My mother had one and I wondered what she had gone through.

Mastectomy is surgery to remove breast tissue from a breast. It used to be that surgeons almost always performed a radical mastectomy, but there have been improvements to the procedure over the last twenty years.

Today, how the mastectomy is performed depends on the factors in the case. Age, general health, menopause status, tumor size and grade, the hormone receptor status, and whether or not the cancer has metastasized are all considered when deciding how to proceed.

After removing tissue, the surgeon can reconstruct the breast, sometimes during the surgery, sometimes later. They can even make a new breast out of basically nothing. Reconstruction uses an implant, tissue from another part of the body, or a combination of both.

Surprise, surprise, a lumpectomy is considered a partial mastectomy. They just don't call it a mastectomy, probably to avoid confusion. When they call it a partial mastectomy rather than a lumpectomy, it is because the surgeon removed more tissue. Reconstruction of the breast may or may not be needed. When they do it, think of it as re-stuffing the existing pillow after some of the stuffing is removed.

A partial radical mastectomy (also called a simple or total mastectomy) removes the whole breast. The skin and the pectoral muscle stay where they belong. This surgery is often performed on women with multiple DCIS tumors and for women who are trying to prevent getting breast cancer. Yes, they can reconstruct the breast.

A modified radical mastectomy takes out the breast and however many lymph nodes. This is the surgery used to treat most invasive tumors. The surgeon can do reconstruction.

Skin sparing mastectomy takes off the nipple, areola, and the original biopsy scar, leaving as much of the skin as possible in order to allow for a more successful reconstruction. Breast tissue is removed through the small(er) opening that is created. The surgeon won't do this if there is a chance there are cancer cells close to the skin. Also, if reconstruction isn't going to happen immediately, he won't want to do this. If you don't have skin saving surgery, the surgeon generally leaves just enough skin to make your chest and scar flat.

A subcutaneous mastectomy spares the nipple. It isn't done often because tissue can be left that might grow tumors. Also, breast reconstruction might not work; this form of mastectomy can cause distortion and numbness of the nipple.

A radical mastectomy is what it always has been: complete removal of the breast, including the nipple. The overlying skin, the muscles underneath the breast, and the lymph nodes on that side of the body are removed. They don't do this so much anymore. It is considered overkill because a partial radical mastectomy is usually as effective and less disfiguring.

The more tissue the surgeon takes out, the more major the surgery. You might stay in the hospital a couple of days; there will be bandages, stitches (probably the type that dissolve) and perhaps a higher degree of difficulty moving your arm.

You might have drains (tubes) to collect the gunk that accumulates in the emptied space. The drains have bulbs to suction out the fluid (think of a turkey baster and you have the idea.) They might or might not be removed before you go home.

The more tissue is removed, the longer recovery takes. Plan on up to a couple of weeks to bounce back from the surgery. You won't be able to wear a bra right away. You might have what they call phantom sensations for a couple of months. It is described as a weird crawly sensation, itching, sensitivity, or pressure because cut nerves have to regrow. And you may have to exercise your arm so you don't stiffen up and lose range of motion.

The more tissue removed, the greater the risk of infection. Sometimes the blood supply to the area is lessened so that healing is delayed. Also, scar tissue can be a problem.

And mastectomy doesn't automatically mean you don't need radiation or chemotherapy.

Wednesday, November 23, 2011

My stomach announced this was to be an eventful day. It was knotted up again, but not as much as other times. I was almost accustomed to the awful feeling.

First, Rick and I took him to the dentist, who had strict orders to have Rick out of the office by 9:45 so we could get to Dr. Chirurgus' office on time. Thank you, Dr. Dentarius, for doing so. We were off to the Lakeside branch of Henry Ford for my surgical follow-up visit and we were on time.

I had three objectives for this medical visit: check that the lumpectomy was successful, find out the pathology of my tumor, and get the damn bandage off. I would slay Dr. Chirurgus if it didn't get removed.

Rick asked if I wanted him in the examining room. Of course I did. When we were called in, he took the chair Martha had used. With a sense of déjà vu, I put on a hospital gown again, not because if flattered my figure. Connie, the so-helpful nurse, was on vacation, visiting her daughter in California. Does everyone have a daughter in California? We should move Michigan closer to the west coast.

A nurse removed the bandage. She guessed the powder on my chest came from surgical gloves. She also commented on the amount of tape involved in my bandage; evidently different nurses use varying amounts of the lethal stuff to glue the bandage to one's breast and mine did a thorough job of it. The nurse gently tugged it off from various directions—so gently that I finally said she might as well rip away. She did and it hurt. She informed me of the broken blister on my back from the tape pulling on my skin. No wonder I itched so much.

Then she lightly scrubbed the left over glue off my skin using their special brand of Goo Gone. Once she was done, Dr. Chirurgus came in.

He checked my breast, handed me a copy of the pathology report and pointed out that the biopsies of both lymph nodes proved benign. I asked if that meant the cancer had not spread and was told that there was virtually no chance of it.

He would like me to schedule another visit with him in six months. Also, I should have a mammogram of the left breast done in six months. This was the culmination of the surgeon's time with me. I wanted to go over the pathology report with him in detail, but he was uncommunicative. No sitting down to discuss it. No detailed information about the lumpectomy. Did he get good clear margins? Yes, but that was all he said. He stood near the door, answered my questions as succinctly as possible (which translates to as briefly as possible) and left in a hurry. The nurse went with him.

What the hell? They didn't even tell me when I could shower, raise my arm, carry anything heavy. Nothing, nada. It was a 180° change from my other meeting with him. Thinking about it, the only thing that made sense was that the doctor had trouble dealing with problems and my skin was a problem. Well, bully for him. I got dressed and we left.

At home, I looked up what to do after lumpectomy. Take sponge baths only until any drains and stitches are taken out. Then you can take a shower. Wait for healing or your doctor's nod before you take a bath. A good support or sports bra worn day and night will help with bothersome movement. Try sleeping on your side with the sore breast closest to the mattress with a pillow under it. If your doctor says, start doing arm exercises the day after surgery.

It was mostly common sense. I could do that.

We were hungry, so Rick and I went to Big Boy Restaurant. Not exciting gourmet food, but reliable. My skin was sore; I was uncomfortable. In the car, I flipped through the pathology report. Mumbo jumbo scientific stuff—stuff easily explained by a doctor. I'd have to hit the Internet again.

We rejoiced that the lymph nodes were clear and puzzled over the pathology report. Not able to interpret it, I set the papers aside to eat.

Tomorrow was Thanksgiving; we could go to the specialty grocery store and get the fresh goods we needed. Potatoes, butternut squash, onions, things like that. Yummy things.

So we went shopping. My skin was going beyond sore and into pain. The underside of my breast and the skin on my stomach were fiery; it was one of the quickest visits to Nino Salvaggio's Fruit Market I ever made. And possibly the cheapest. I didn't get any fresh cheese, we didn't browse for dessert stuff. We got the minimum we needed to produce Thanksgiving dinner and left. By the time we got home, I was desperate to do something about my skin. I was at the end of my rope.

Rick unloaded the car—three measly bags of groceries—while I headed for the bedroom and the pack of Olay wipes. The cool, smooth wet cloth eased the burn, at least for a while. I next took a pain pill. Was I at the end of my rope? Yes, and someone hacked it off. With the rope hanging limp in my hand, I couldn't even get up the gumption to take a shower. I hurt as badly as the day of the lumpectomy—more.

Later, I took a shower, but couldn't bear to use soap on my skin. The water stung. A lavish application of Eucerin made life bearable. It must have been the Goo Gone irritating my skin. Why did I keep forgetting it was sensitive? Get it in gear, Ann.

One side effect you may have after surgery is blood clots forming either under your breast or in the armpit. This is Mondor's Disease. No, it's not a disease—Henri Mondor just named it that way. It is actually thrombophlebitis (inflammation) of the superficial veins. The area affected will hurt a little, swell a little, and turn a little red. It is usually mild and will clear itself up. A warm compress and over-the-counter pain reliever should be sufficient to provide relief. Nope, it didn't happen to me.

Friday, November 25, 2011

Taking pain pills on a regular schedule (and not telling Rick I was taking them,) I managed to cook a Thanksgiving feast. Rick was a trooper as sous chef. Thanks to watching the Food Channel, he changed how he carved the turkey. Thanks to watching the Food Channel, I had two new recipes to try. One for butternut squash, which I have never succeeded in cooking well, and the other for roasted Brussels sprouts. My family cannot understand why I adore Brussels sprouts.

Sad to say, it was not the most successful Thanksgiving. The turkey was dry, the dressing had crisp bits of bread all over, and I burned the brussels sprouts so much even I didn't like them. But I pulled dinner off with the assistance of my willing sous chef, who deserved a bonus, only forgetting to use salt and pepper in the mashed potatoes. The squash was a hit.

Then I had the luxury of examining my skin. Oh, lord, what a mess. On my back, right where a bra cuts, was a two inch oval blister missing its protective skin covering. That was what had itched so much. In an arc under my arm was a red line directing attention to a 2x2 inch square of suture tape where the lymph nodes were removed. (No stitches. They used this special tape that acts as stitches.) The square didn't hurt, but the tape was starting to curl and was scratchy on my arm. Underneath my breast, on my stomach, was a vividly square patch of skin that looked like one whale of a sunburn. There was a matching area of redness on the underside of my breast. The patches were up close and personal with each other. The seam where breast meets chest, between the two distressed areas, was scarlet. Just looking, you would know that it HURT.

A decent distance up the slope of my breast from the redness was a curved four inch incision. That was the lumpectomy site. It was covered by a string of more surgical tape, mostly neat and tidy, but beginning to come loose at the lower end. The incision was sensitive at the top edge, where one could see a slight seepage of blood, but the tape was holding things together nicely.

The top of my breast was in the best shape; that skin spends time in the sun and is less delicate. No wonder I was cranky. I had not donned a bra since Lumpectomy Day and there was no way I was wearing one until my skin healed. And now I knew I had trouble with surgical tape.

This was partially my fault. I knew my skin tended to be sensitive; I knew I had problems with band-aids. I should have told Dr. Chirurgus, but I forgot. To be honest, I never thought about surgical bandages in the context of lumpectomies.

The thing about 4 and 5 o'clock was right. Flatten my boob, paste clock numerals on, and the incision was between 4 and 5.

Let's move along from transitory discomfort. I had a surgical report to dissect. If he failed at communication, at least the surgeon gave me the pathology report.

I didn't have a prayer of deciphering it without the help of the Internet. Without the hours spent searching, I would have missed some very important points.

The Pathology Report

The first page had the Pathological Diagnosis:
A. Left axillary sentinel lymph node 1, biopsy:
   Benign lymph node, one.
B. Left axillary sentinel lymph node 2, biopsy:
   Benign lymph node, one.

Joy to the world. There was no cancer in the lymph nodes. One of my hurdles passed with flying colors.

There was a gross description of the lymph nodes. One was gray white, the other gray white to yellow lobular homogenous, whatever that means. From information off the Internet, the gross descriptions are not significant—they are just impressions of what the pathologist sees. Then there was a full page of stains, blocks, and comments about charged slides. Total mumbo jumbo. It appeared to be notes on the microscopic examination of the nodes.

Page three of the report had the nitty gritty information. It was the Pathologic Diagnosis of left breast, excision with localization (excision meaning it was cut out, localization being the wires stuck in to guide the surgeon.) Then it gave the diagnosis. "Invasive ductal carcinoma, moderately differentiated, margins negative, see synoptic report." This was not news. I already knew the first part. The "margins negative" meant that the surgeon managed to dig out the tumors with enough surrounding them that the pathologist was satisfied he got it all. Good.

I flipped through, but there were no synoptic reports.

The second line said "Ductal carcinoma in situ (DCIS,) high grade, margins negative." This was the second tumor, the one found by MRI. In situ means it was trapped in the milk duct—nothing had gotten out. That was more good news, that it was in the duct, with no little bits wandering around. It was noninvasive (not spreading around,) though it could have turned invasive.

High grade—what did that mean? Well, it turns out they rate DCIS much the same way they rate Invasive Ductal Carcinoma. It's a scale—Low, Medium, and High. Low means the cells look pretty normal. Medium has the cells looking weirder and growing more rapidly. High—the type I had—is cells gone wild. As breastcancer.org says, "People with high-grade DCIS have a higher risk of invasive cancer, either when the DCIS is diagnosed or at some point in the future. They also have an increased risk of the cancer coming back earlier—within the first 5 years rather than after 5 years." High grade poses a greater risk. Ain't life grand.

Right off the bat, I had questions for the doctors:
- Was the DCIS being tested for hormone receptors?
- Was it connected to the other tumor?
- Did it add anything to or change the treatment plan?

Okay, back to the pathology report. The rest of it applied only to the invasive carcinoma—the first tumor, the one found by mammogram. Right away, I had to do more research on the Internet because we had gotten to Histologic grade, which had numbers. I didn't know what the numbers meant.

Here is what my report said:

Histologic grade

Tubule formation: 2 Moderate (10-75%)
Tubule score: 2
Nuclear pleomorphism: 2
Moderate increase in size etc.
Nuclear score: 2
Mitotic count: 3
Greater than 10 mitoses per 10 HPF
Mitotic score: 3
Total Nottingham score:
G2, Moderately differentiated (6-7 points)
Total score: 7

Eek. We have to get really technical here. The Abramson Cancer Center of the University of Pennsylvania obligingly spelled it out. Let's go line by line, starting with a brief explanation.

It's known as the Nottingham style of classifying tumors. The Center says, "It is a combination of nuclear grade, mitotic rate, and tubule formation, which are characteristics of the tumor cells seen under a microscope that predict its aggressiveness. Now, this scoring system is very detailed and usually does not affect treatment decisions, so it is not particularly helpful in the big picture." Which isn't to say that I didn't care. Each element is scored using a scale of 1 to 3, with one being nicest and three nastiest.

The first score is Tubule formation. The pathologist looks at the tumor through a microscope and figures out how many of the cancer cells are in a tubular shape. How many of them look like manicotti pasta? The more the merrier, so a score of 1 means you have lots of manicotti. My score was 2, in the middle. Some manicotti, some something else. Macaroni? Shells?

Nuclear pleomorphism tells what the center of the cancer cells look like. 1 means they look pretty darn normal. Again, my score was 2, in the middle.

Mitotic count is how fast the cells are multiplying. A score of 1 means the tumor is lazy. My score was 3, the fastest growing.

To come up with the Nottingham score, those three numbers are added together. The lowest total possible is 3 and the highest is 9. For low grade, you need a score 3-5, medium grade 6-7, high grade 8-9. At least in theory, the higher the number you end up with, the nastier the cancer you are dealing with. I had a score of 7, high middle grade. I was not too happy with that score. Hurdle-wise, I stubbed my toe but good.

Research on the Internet is both curse and blessing. Working to understand the Nottingham score, I found researchers who think the most critical component of the score is the Mitotic count. If you have a higher score for the Mitotic count, your tumor is more dangerous. It is more difficult to get rid of; it comes back more often. The other two parts of the Nottingham score don't matter as much for predicting the course of a cancer. Curses on the Internet; ignorance would be bliss. Dangerous, but blissful.

Back to the pathology report. The MIB-1 or ki-67 immunostain was positive with strong intensity in 50-60% of tumor cells. Ki-67 is a tumor marker; the higher the percentage, the faster growing the tumor. It meant that when they tested my tumor, 50-60% of the cells were actively growing—a sign of higher malignancy. This can perhaps be used to estimate the outcome of the cancer battle; if it grows really fast, it metastasizes faster. But if the percentage is higher, chemotherapy is more effective against it. Evidently, some studies have decided that a high ki-67 number is bad for survival, and others that it makes no difference. I did find mention on the Internet that if your tumor is triple negative to expect a ki-67 between 50 and 90, so mine was on the lower end of what I could expect.

This was one time when my oncologists failed me. With all my questioning, all my demands to be told the full truth, they never told me my tumors were fast growing. I never found out if they were like basal cells. I can understand the doctors' reticence—they didn't want to scare me. They didn't want to discourage me. Only God would help me if I gave up the fight. But I don't do well with uncertainty. I would have liked to KNOW.

The next line of the pathology reports told me that the maximum dimension of my tumor was 1.6 centimeters. What? My tumor was measured in millimeters: 6x9x4. Now it was lots bigger. Did it grow that fast? There was another question for the doctors.

Then the report gave details of the margins around the junk they dug out of my breast. For the invasive tumor, it was about 0.1 centimeters. For the DCIS, it was 0.15 centimeters. This was important because I wanted the surgeon to have melon balled out all of the cancer cells. If the margins were clean, it was more likely they got everything.

But how large did the margin need to be? The Abramson Cancer Center said 1-2 millimeters was considered standard. Now I had to do the math. How many millimeters are there in a centimeter? Answer: 10 millimeters. So, the margin around my invasive tumor was 1 millimeter, 1½ millimeters for the DCIS. Acceptable to pathologists. Why did I wish they had gotten a bit more? Maybe a centimeter more?

Extensive intraductal component (EIC) was the next item in the list. One would have a positive response on the pathology report if 25% or more of the invasive breast cancer consists of intraductal carcinoma (another term for DCIS,) while ductal carcinoma in situ (DCIS) is also present as a second spot. Boiling it down to plain English, do you have two tumors? If so, is one DCIS and the other at least 25% DCIS cells? Does the second tumor appear to have been DCIS at an earlier time? It matters because it is another predictor of cancer behavior. My pathology report said I didn't have it, but I wondered if the size of my tumor influenced the negative response. So, it was another question for the doctors.

The pathology report went on to mention angiolymphatic invasion, which I didn't have. If I did, the cancer cells would be actively trying to get to the bloodstream, where they might take a free ride to other sites. Hurrah, some good news.

Dermal lymphatic invasion is when the tumor has gotten to the skin. No, I didn't have it.

The report promised that tests had been ordered to determine breast tumor markers as well as estrogen, progesterone and Her-2/neu status. Breast tumor markers are signs, generally proteins that show up in your blood, when you have cancer. I didn't know what they might be looking for, so I added that to my questions.

The estrogen, progesterone and Her-2/neu receptors were already known for the invasive tumor; was this testing for the second tumor? My, I was going to have plenty of questions for the doctor.

According to the next line in the pathology report, my primary tumor was pT1c, greater than 1 centimeter but not greater than 2 centimeters in greatest dimension. I couldn't find an exact explanation, only a doctor answering a question on the Internet said pT1c meant the third part of Stage I with no lymph node involvement. Finally, I found a chart.

pT refers to the primary tumor. The number indicates the size of the tumor and how far it has spread:

Stage 0		abnormal cells in the duct (DCIS,) but they are not cancerous. They could become cancerous
Stage I	pTis	stuck in the duct
	pT1	20 mm or smaller
	pT1m	1 mm or smaller
	pT1a	1-5 mm
	pT1b	6-10 mm
	pT1c	larger than 1 cm but smaller than 2 cm
Stage II	pT2	2-5 cm
Stage III	pT3	bigger than 5 cm
Stage IV	pT4	doesn't matter what size it is, it has reached the chest wall and/or the skin

There are more criteria involved in assigning the number. For example, there are more numbers if lymph nodes are involved or if the cancer has spread another way.

There are four possible stages, with one being the best and four the most lethal. The stage is simply how advanced the tumor is. Stage IV means you are in a serious fight for survival. Just don't let it panic you. People can and have survived Stage IV cancer.

The last two lines of the page were for lymph nodes and distant metastasis. Both said they could not be assessed, which added them to my list of questions.

The next page of the report gave the gross description of the mass Dr. Chirurgus pulled out of my breast. Other than being a tan-white ill-defined mass, in size it was 6.5 x 5.5 x 3.5 centimeters (roughly 2½ inches by 2 inches by 1½ inches.) The tumor was 1.6 x 1.2 x .8 centimeters (more than a half an inch by less than a half of an inch by a third of an inch,) so it sounded like it must have lots of little seed cells floating around it. I would ask the doctor.

What I most wished to ask about was, "There are small two minute nodules 1.2 centimeters anterolaterally to mass." What did that mean? Did I have little spots of cancer all over the place?

I was scheduled to see the oncology doctor in charge of chemotherapy on Monday. I hoped she scheduled time to go over this mess with me.

Let's backtrack a moment and address an issue I ignored because it didn't happen to me. When lymph nodes are removed, no matter how few or how many, one has to become aware of a possible side effect of that removal: a condition called Lymphedema (everyone misspells it as lymphodemia.) It is swelling caused by poor circulation of lymph fluid.

Losing those lymph nodes can be a real pain in the patootie; the drainage system can get fouled and the fluid backs up, just like when your sewer backs up into your basement. The liquid has to go somewhere. It sits in your basement and ruins your box of photos or it backs up into your arm and hand, swelling you up. And like cleaning your basement, getting the fluid out isn't easy. It is much easier to avoid the problem in the first place.

The first defense against Lymphedema is never have your blood pressure taken via the arm on the side of the missing nodes. Also, forget having blood drawn from that side… or getting shots in that arm… watch for infection… don't sling a heavy purse from that shoulder. Don't do things to upset that arm.

I've seen pictures of women with Lymphedema. Their hands and arms swell (sometimes elsewhere,) making clothing fit poorly, making them miserable. Evidently, once it gets going, there is no cure for evil sidekick Lymphedema, only ways to handle it. One way is to wear a compression bandage on the arm. It would squeeze the fluid back up, away from the hand. They are not comfortable, but if you need them, you need them. Physical therapy might be called for.

You certainly don't want to ignore swelling.

Lymphedema is not a foregone conclusion. My mother, for one, lost all the lymph nodes on one side of her body and never developed it. But there is no sense tempting fate. I was very good at reminding nurses which arm they could work on. Every once in a while a nurse would forget and head for the side that was missing lymph nodes; I would cheerfully head her in the right direction.

It's my body. Ultimately, I am the one responsible for it.

It's time for a little inspiration

You gain strength, courage, and confidence by every experience in which you really stop to look fear in the face. *Eleanor Roosevelt*

Strength does not come from physical capacity. It comes from an indomitable will. *Mahatma Gandhi*

You can be a victim of cancer or a survivor of cancer. It's a mindset. *Dave Pelzer*

No one saves us but ourselves. No one can and no one may. We ourselves must walk the path. *Buddha*

Chemotherapy

Monday, November 28, 2011

Today I saw the chemotherapy oncologist, Dr. Medica. Rick accompanied me. His manager, Tom, told him to do what he had to do and Rick chose to support me. I suggested he go to work for a couple of hours; I would pick him up for the appointment. When we were done, he could go back.

I drove Martha to work and had well over an hour before I had to pick Rick up, so I took myself to Farmer's Restaurant in Eastern Market. Truckers eat there. Any place truckers eat has good food. I had a book in my purse to enjoy while I ate an omelet. Then it was time to collect Rick and head for the hospital.

Rick was prompt; we shot up the expressway and found the Clinic entrance on the side of the hospital. By the time we got to the waiting room, we had a fifteen minute wait until my 10:30 appointment. I signed in, we sat, and I decided to go to the bathroom, which didn't take long. When I came back, they had called for me. The nurse was going to return. Doesn't that figure?

In a few minutes, the nurse came back to get us. I got weighed; it was rock steady, even with all the cheesecake I had been eating since Thanksgiving, then we waited in the hall to find out which examining room we were to use. Someone had snitched Dr. Medica's room. She insists on using the rooms with windows. I don't know, maybe she is claustrophobic.

Before we saw Dr. Medica, we saw a medical student, Andy. Lordy, they make them young, although he probably wasn't as youthful as he looked. Like my daughters, he would have trouble looking like a full grown adult well into his thirties. But he was nice, not at all lofty. He wanted to be a children's oncologist.

He had questions; I answered, but they were not critical. I bet he was working on his bedside manner. I decided to give him something to do; I handed him my questions from the pathology report and asked if he could answer any. He tried, but I don't think he was permitted to get technical. He didn't get down to the meat of the questions.

Then the oncologist, Dr. Medica, came in, a small woman with over the shoulder fly-away hair, and a soft, accented voice. She impressed me because not once did I have the urge to contradict her. She didn't make mistakes. She was competent. I trusted her.

This mattered. I guess you could say I mistrust authority. In high school I talked back to teachers, vocally disagreeing with them, even if it got me in trouble. I was snippy to a police officer when he repeatedly thought my last name (Tracy) was my first name. I'll argue with the mayor during city council meetings without a second thought. No, I am not intimidated by authority, and I don't have any compunction questioning authority figures. Dr. Medica didn't bring this out in me.

Along with her examining my poor abused skin and breast, feeling lymph nodes, and checking my belly (for constipation, I think,) I gave Dr. Medica my questions. She didn't have the pathology report; she sent someone to retrieve a copy, and we got along with our business.

Our dealings took three and a half hours, so don't expect a minute accounting. Better, let's get done with the pathology report before we get into the fascinating topic of chemotherapy.

These are the questions with Dr. Medica's answers:
- Was the DCIS connected to the other tumor?
  Answer: Who knows which grew first? No, they didn't consider them connected.
- Did it add anything to or change the treatment plans?
  Answer: There was no change in my treatment plan after the decision to add chemotherapy.
- Maximum dimension of the tumor was 1.6 centimeters. No, my tumor was measured in millimeters: 6x9x4. Now it was lots larger. Did it grow that fast?
  Answer: The millimeter size was what they snipped out for the biopsy. (Why didn't anyone tell me that before?) Mammograms and MRIs can't be as accurate as actually playing with the tumors, so predicting the size is not exact. The DCIS was actually larger than the invasive tumor. I was Stage I... enough. And my mind flitted back to the doctor who gave me the diagnosis. She had said "advanced stage" and size-wise, she had been somewhat right. It was working toward a more advanced tumor in size. I had gotten lucky that everything else about it was firmly Stage I.

- Extensive intraductal component—was the size of my tumor influencing the negative response? If the tumor was smaller, would the answer be yes?
  Answer: Dr. Medica said straight out that it didn't matter. Not important, folks.
- Breast tumor markers —what were they?
  Answer: She wanted a baseline of my breast tumor markers, which are proteins floating around in my blood that indicate cancer. The baseline would be used in the future to help watch for a recurrence of cancer.
- Estrogen, progesterone and Her-2/neu receptors—retesting the invasive tumor or testing the DCIS?
  Answer: She didn't know what was being tested, but would find out.
- Lymph nodes and distant metastasis could not be assessed?
  Answer: Meaningless in my case. Ignore, ignore.
- There were small two minute nodules 1.2 centimeters anterolaterally to mass. What did that mean? Did I have little spots of cancer other than what was removed?

This question gave Dr. Medica pause. She did not know what it meant on the pathology report, but she intended to find out. Speaking to medical student Andy, she explained why it might matter. Divide the breast into quarters: having two or more tumors in two or more quarters gives a different character to cancer—it is treated differently. Having one or two tumors in one quarter is not significant, but if there are more clustered together then treatment maybe should be reevaluated.

Think of it like ants. If you see three or four tiny ants marching across your kitchen floor, get out the broom and then wash the floor and maybe set out an ant trap. The ants have smelled food; close their restaurant and they will go elsewhere. But if you see three or four ants in the kitchen and six in the bathroom, call the Orkin Man. It's an invasion.

It was reassuring to know Dr. Medica was going to check. Maybe I should be concerned that she had not seen the full surgical pathology report, but then again, why would she need to? She handles chemotherapy and in theory knew everything she needed to know to plan the attack. (Actually, I believe treatment plans are made in committee meetings. Probably the guy who knows what the pathology report says tells everyone the important info and then they all decide what should be done.)

The surprise here was that I should aim for a two year survival rate. No, I was not going to die; as far as I could tell, I was nowhere near dying.

But I found the information on the Internet and I asked Dr. Medica if it was true.

She informed me that the type of cancer I had was likely to recur within two years. Every year I got past the two year mark without a recurrence of the cancer, the better my chances got. The trick was destroying all the cancer cells. Leave a few in, and it would come back. No ifs here. The longer I got past two years without the cancer popping back up, the more likely it was gone for good. Pass that mark, celebrate, and then aim for five years. We didn't discuss percentages. She did tell me that if I reached five years without a recurrence, she would consider me cured.

Damn it, Cancer, you are not going to get me. I am not going to die from you. Do you hear? I mean it from the bottom of my soul. We have a plan of attack, not seat of the pants ramblings.

Dr. Medica chose for me to have six courses or cycles (six times) of TC chemotherapy. TC stands for Taxotere and Cyclophosphamide, two different drugs that prevent cancer cells from dividing (growing) and eventually (hopefully) make them shrink and die. It is a standard menu, but usually given four times, not six. I was favored with two additional treatments because I was triple negative. It was rigorous treatment, she told me.

I would have a port in my chest; a semi-permanent IV thing, because the veins in my arms wouldn't tolerate the drugs going in through them.

She started to list the most common side effects of chemotherapy, and I mentioned that I hoped to lose my appetite, and thus shed some weight. No, the treatments tend to make people hungry, so weight gain was common. For heaven's sake, I got cancer and would get fatter? Andy suggested a wasting disease like Tuberculosis, and Dr. Medica winced. I loved Andy's bedside manner; someday a bunch of kids might feel a little better because of his sense of humor. I offered him one of my daughters to marry and he regretfully declined.

Oh well, gaining weight would be nasty, but I was trying to be realistic. I would rather be fatter and alive than skinnier and dead. Ideally, I would be as thin as I was in high school and brimming with health. Get real.

There were zillions of side effects, only a couple of which were truly dire. The horrible ones were:

Allergic reaction. Anyone with any sense knows that allergic reactions can be bad. A reaction was more common with the first or second dose of TC. If I started to have trouble breathing, I should head for the emergency room. Anything less awful, like hives or another rash, swelling (unless it was near my throat,) itching, or flushing, I should call Dr. Medica.

Neuropathy. It is damage to nerves from the chemicals. I should be most aware of tingling or numbness in fingers or toes and report it immediately, as there were things that could be done to help. It was most apt to happen right after a chemo dose and hopefully was temporary. I did need to be aware that neuropathy can be permanent.

My friendly Internet told me in more detail what Dr. Medica told me: certain chemotherapy drugs can cause peripheral (around the edges) neuropathy (nerve damage,) most commonly in fingers and toes, but also in the bowel, causing constipation and even intestinal blockage, or to the face, back or chest. The symptoms run from numbness and tingling, weakness, pain, burning, loss of sensation, to losing touch with a part of your body. Cross your fingers, folks. I was not anxious to deal with neuropathy.

If my liver was weak (which it wasn't,) chemo could mess it up more. It could do nasty things to my skin, but that doesn't happen often. It could cause bleeding in the bladder. Don't forget the lungs; chemo could mess with them also, even scarring them. If I had no luck whatsoever, the Cyclophosphamide could cause more cancer or leukemia sometime down the road.

Water retention and delayed wound healing sounded like lesser evils here, but they were also side effects of the drugs. Losing my hair was inevitable; it should grow back, but I disliked the thought of losing my eyebrows and eyelashes more than what was on my head and legs.

Chemo drugs make one's eyes water, but to avoid a narrowing of the tear ducts, I should use a good eye drop, like Refresh, frequently. It would help flush the drugs out of my eyes. Also, drink lots and lots of water to flush the drugs out of my body.

Keep in mind that chemotherapy has an endless list of side effects. The reason is that chemo trashes your immune system. It is poison used to treat a killer. It attacks healthy parts of your body. In order to banish the dreaded hooded guy with a scythe, you risk other problems. Chemo is not really optional; you have to have it. What is the alternative? Almost certain death.

I was supposed to call in if I had:
- Shaking chills or fever of 100.5° F or higher
- Unusual bleeding, easy bruising, or pinpoint red spots on the skin
- Vomiting that is severe or that lasts several hours
- Painful or frequent urination or blood in the urine
- Diarrhea that causes an additional four bowel movements a day, diarrhea that lasts more than one day, diarrhea at night or diarrhea with fever, cramps, or bloody stools

- Irregular or rapid heartbeat, chest pain, chest tightness, or shortness of breath
- Dizziness or feeling lightheaded
- Inability to eat or weight loss
- Pain or blisters in the mouth, stomach, or genitals
- Swelling around the eyes
- Pain in the arms or legs
- Sudden shortness of breath

This was encouraging, wasn't it?

The good news was that they would give me stuff before and after the treatments to handle some of the common side effects. I should expect to feel poorly for a few days after each treatment and then improve. And while the treatments hit people differently, I heard about one lady who went out to lunch after every chemo treatment. Maybe I would be one of the lucky ones.

A Clinical Trial

Dr. Medica offered for me to join a clinical trial. What is a clinical trial? It is research that has gone from theoretical (someone's good idea) to being tested. It passed the stage of being inflicted on white mice or rats so successfully that the government has said they can do it on me, if I agree. The trial Dr. Medica was interested in was nothing so very radical; it added a common cancer drug, Herceptin (AKA Trastuzumab,) to my treatment.

As Dr. Medica explained, Herceptin is given to people with Her-2/neu positive tumors, but when researchers went back and checked, some of those people turned out to be Her-2/neu negative. Herceptin seemed to help them be cured. Why? The thought is this:

Cancer is composed of a bunch of cells, not just one. What if some of those cells are Her-2/neu negative and some are Her-2/neu positive? When a tumor is checked for Her-2/neu, it can have a score of +1, +2, or +3. Three is positive. One (and I think two) is negative. Since even negative tumors can show a little bit of Her-2/neu positive qualities, the hope is that the clinical trial will figure out if Herceptin helps Her-2/neu negative tumors die by killing Her-2/neu positive cells in it.

My tumor was +1, so I was the highest possible Her-2/neu negative. The TC drugs were designed to fight Her-2/neu negative cancers. It wouldn't touch any Her-2/neu positive cells in my tumors. We might be merrily killing three quarters or nine tenths of my tumor and letting the rest get off scot free, ready, willing and able to keep growing and kill me.

The trial could be a winning situation for me—it could kill Her-2/neu positive cells in my tumors. That would be good.

Then again, the trial might not do anything. There were two ways it could be useless:

1) As a white mouse in the clinical trial, I might not get the drug. If I didn't get it, I would be a control subject, one of the people they used to measure other people's success by. I would be helping researchers learn how to better deal with cancer, but I would not benefit myself.
2) As a white mouse in the clinical trial, I might get Herceptin, but it might not help me. The idea they are testing might be wrong, or Herceptin might not be a good way to deal with the problem. God forbid, it might even be harmful to me, but I think they would pull me out of the study if they could tell it was hurting me.

The important point was I would not get Herceptin unless I joined the clinical trial. The government had not authorized its use for my type of cancer.

What did I have to lose? I promised myself that I would do whatever I had to do, however distasteful, disgusting, or distressing, in order to be cured of cancer. Joining the clinical trial added more drugs, more tests, more side effects, more danger, more fuss, muss, to do, and effort to my plate. It would mean ten years of greater and lesser involvement with the medical community before the trial ended.

Was it worth it? Yes. I signed up for the clinical trial.

Rick, who had been a quiet presence all this time, had a question. Should we stick with our current Blue Cross insurance, which was a good plan, but had high deductibles, or should he switch us to HAP (Health Alliance Plan?) The doctor sent the lady in charge of billing to talk to us.

HAP, an HMO, is a part of the Henry Ford Health System. As long as we stayed with Henry Ford Health System doctors, etc., we should have no problems. If the doctors wanted to do something that was not covered, they would argue it out with HAP; billing lady had not run into a situation which was not successfully covered. The deductibles and co-pays were miniscule compared to Blue Cross and that was the deciding factor. We didn't have a burning desire to go bankrupt making me healthy. We owed over $400 for the MRI; our bills were nearing the $4,200 deductible for 2011 as we spoke. How could we add another $4,200 bill to our budget next year?

Rick would switch us to HAP.

The last person we talked to was Trish, a Clinical Research Coordinator.

I liked her immediately. I didn't know what her other duties might be in the Clinical Trials Office, but she promised to be my personal secretary and sounding board. If I needed something, even just a shoulder to cry on, I should call her. Not at 3 am—she wouldn't answer the phone. She would coordinate my appointments; she would remind me what drugs to take and when to take them. She probably should have Martha's email address. Martha is permanently connected to her email account through her phone, which never turns off and seldom leaves her side, so if Trish needed to tell me something, Martha was a sure bet to get through to me. If I couldn't be found, Martha would find me.

Let me put it this way. I don't like phones. I have a cell phone that lives in my purse. If it has power, if is turned on, if I hear it ring, and if the call is from Katie, Rick, or Martha, I will answer it. In other words, don't call my cell phone. The land line at home is answered if I am home and hear it ring unless the call appears to be telemarketing. If Katie, Rick, or Martha calls, I definitely answer unless I am asleep (though sometimes I answer and promptly forget after I fall back asleep) or can't get to it, in which case I check to see who called.

I don't slavishly check my email either. Yes, Trish should have Martha's contact information.

The last person I saw was the girl who draws blood. She wanted two vials, please. Then Rick and I were out of there. It was 2 pm; he was starving and I was hungry. He needed to run home and get his keys, which he forgot this morning and then he needed to go to work.

We went to Janet's for a burger; Jerry was there. He was getting up to leave when we entered. Bless his teddy bear soul, he stayed until we left. I called Martha and told her Dad would have the car and Rick took me home.

Home again, home again, jiggedy jog.

Tuesday, November 29, 2011

Yesterday was such a drawn out process, I thought today would be a break. No. Henry Ford called. Could I please have more blood drawn tomorrow? Yes, I'd go to Cottage Hospital.

Henry Ford called. Let's schedule the echocardiogram, a requirement of the clinical trial, if not of Dr. Medica. Ok, December 6th. At Cottage Hospital again.

Henry Ford called. They want to insert the port in my chest. Can we do it December 7th? She would email me the instructions. Someone would have to take me to Henry Ford Hospital and drive me home. I would be there about four hours.

Henry Ford called. They phoned in a prescription to the pharmacy for the skin under my breast, which looked like it might be thinking of starting a yeast infection.

My daughter told me that the complexity of my treatment threw me into a management team's inbox. The calls were them making sure things got done as they reviewed my file.

I was now eligible to be tested for the bad genes that cause cancer. I made an appointment at the genetics place.

Some people (Hah. Lots of people) are afraid of medical tests. Does a needle make you sweat? Are you claustrophobic in the PET scanner? Scared of being put to sleep? There are ways to deal with anxiety.

First, tell the test giver you are scared. They should take their time, explain what they are doing—or rush through it, talking about the latest Hollywood scandal, if that is easier for you.

It's not shameful to ask for a tranquilizer if it will get you over the hump.

There are more creative ways to deal with fear. Imagine you are on a beach—or accepting that $10 million lottery winning check. Belt out a song, recite the Declaration of Independence (we have the right to pursue happiness,) plan Christmas dinner down to the color of the napkins...

Anything that works to distract you is acceptable.

Remind yourself, "What is the worst that can happen?" You might have a panic attack or faint. Or have a heart attack, in which case you are in the best place you could be—in front of a medical person who can deal with it. Are you going to see that medical person again? Do you really care what they think? Tell yourself "No" very firmly.

Eat a good meal (at the appropriate time.) Take a walk. Sleep well the night before. Can't sleep? Don't try to nod off; try to stay awake. That might do the trick. Argue with yourself. Promise yourself a reward (and follow through.)

Give yourself good reasons to suffer. Not only are you working to fix your cancer, but you are proving to your ___ that you are ___. Fill in the blanks with something that really matters to you; I suggest mother/third grade teacher/dry cleaners paired with presidential material/ Superwoman/Princess Diana.

Hypnosis might convince you that all is well enough to get through the procedure. Heck, it might pull you through all the tests and procedures coming up.

You could do what I did. I used to be scared of the dentist. Then I got a wicked abscess in my chin. The tooth had calcified (as hard as stone) and the dentist had trouble drilling through it. It took several appointments, and after each appointment, I had a bad toothache. Finally, I told Dr. Dentist to just get it done. I cried as he drilled through that tooth. Dr. Dentist told me he felt like a child abuser, but lo and behold, I lost my fear. I think it was realizing he had already done the worst that could happen, so what more was there to fear?

Don't expect perfection. It's okay to be afraid. What isn't okay is to not go through with the procedure. If all else fails, go ahead and faint. First, tell them to get it done before you wake up.

Thursday, December 1, 2011

There are a couple of medical "housekeeping" chores one should do before starting chemotherapy.

Go to the dentist and get your teeth cleaned, cavities filled, etc. Doing any of this stuff during chemo is well-nigh impossible. Tell Dr. Dentist about your diagnosis and follow his advice.

Make an appointment to visit your eye doctor. If you don't have one, find one. You want to be aware if you have any conditions such as glaucoma or cataracts that could be affected by the coming chemical regimen. You also want someone to check your eyes once or twice during chemo—some sad things could happen that need attending.

Check in with any other doctor you see. A good doctor will want to be in the know and will be aware of any special concerns to watch for. If there are really important/convoluted things involved, the dentist, ophthalmologist, doctor, etc. might want to talk to the oncologist. Chemotherapy hits all parts of your body, not just cancer cells in your breast.

Friday, December 2, 2011

I pulled the last of the surgical tape off the lumpectomy incision. On the upper curve it was stubborn, not curling, not loosening much. The incision had healed, so off it came. The scar from the lumpectomy was not something I ever wanted to show off. Lumpy ugly thing. No one but Rick and doctors would see it, which was fine by me.

Once it was completely healed, I'd massage the scar. That might help smooth it out. Castor oil, vitamin E cream, Aloe Vera, onion extract, Argan oil, Scar Recover Gel, Mederma, Vaseline, or Super Serum Advance+ might make a difference. I guess which worked (if any) depended on the person.

The skin prescription was a powder, Nystatin, that I shook on twice a day. It worked miracles on a yeast infection. No more redness under my breast, no more discomfort, except where I had boo boos from the tape. Those didn't hurt much, so I almost felt on top of the world.

Rick signed us up for HAP.

It rained, and the chimney flashing gave out. I called the roofer recommended by Glenn Haege from The Handyman Show. He had proof of insurance, proof of licensing, samples of shingles, and an understanding heart. If we wanted to beggar ourselves, we could do it right. $10,000 for a nice, new roof. How about if we did a slap dash job? For just under $800, the roofers would peel three roofs (one on top of the other) away from the chimney, install new flashing, and do whatever was needed to make the shingles do their job. I agreed; $800 was less than I thought it would be. Merry Christmas to Rick and myself. Unless Santa did a number on the chimney, the water in the wall would dry up and we (who am I kidding?) Rick could patch and repaint.

There were so many things to do. A laptop and desktop to return to their owners and another desktop came in dead as a doornail. I had to figure out why and fix it if I could.

Henry Ford Health System called while I was out, wanting to schedule a PET scan. They left a message, so I called. The scan had to be done before I started chemo; how about December 7th? No, I was getting the port that day. Even if I wanted to, I couldn't get from the hospital to 15 Mile and Ryan in half an hour—and that was judging times by best case scenario. The next available date was the following Wednesday, at noon. That would work.

For the procedure, a technician would shoot radioactive gunk into me. Then we'd wait for it to wander around my body. Once I was lit up like a virtual Christmas tree, the technician would run me through the scanner and see what, if anything, turned up that looked like cancer. I couldn't help but think it was like putting paper through a computer scanner. Hope they didn't flatten me. The girl would email the directions.

It sounded very high tech, so I went on the Internet to see what I could find out about PET scans. Yep, it's a fancy x-ray machine that can spot malignancies. I guessed it was like a MRI, meaning another round tube that would give me claustrophobic willies. Gack—the things I did to stay alive!

I got the directions for the PET scan via email. No, it was not how to get to the place, but what not to do and what to do. To get ready, I had to eat a low carb diet for 24 hours—they had a detailed menu planned for me, and then nothing except water for 6 hours before the scan. How depressing.

If I took a relaxing Xanax, the scan would see into my body better, so I had to call Henry Ford Health System (Trish) and ask her to prescribe one. Because I was going to take Xanax, they didn't want me to drive, so I had to arrange for Rick or Martha to play chauffeur. The procedure would take about four hours, so that shot the day for my chauffeur.

Because the scan was going to be a week later than they wanted, I called my handy dandy personal secretary, Trish, to let her know of the delay. She ran a couple of other possible dates through her head and agreed that the PET scan would have to be the 14th.

I should have an EKG also; after I had the port put in, could I run up to the 13th floor of the hospital (no, I was doing no marathons on the stairs. I would take the elevator) so Trish could see it got done? I could do that, provided I remembered. I didn't remember to ask for a Xanax. She made a note to give a heads up to someone to steer me in the right direction.

She casually said, "Chemo will have to wait til the next day." I didn't ask Trish to clarify that statement. I was smart enough to figure it out. If no one called to let me know when and where, I would call Trish back. But not now. Enough for today.

My nipple itched, and every once in a while, I got a little twinge in my lumpectomied breast. I didn't feel like calling anyone to ask, and I forgot to mention it to Trish (my memory is a force of nature—oblivious to all prayers and desires,) so I turned once again to the trusty Internet.

The sensations are a part of the healing process. It might be irritated nerves, or severed nerve endings trying to find their other halves, or—this was my thought—it might be the fat shifting around and getting settled.

Me, I felt a little twingey if I slept on my stomach. Some women had sore, hot, swollen breasts, sometimes for months. Evidently, the biggest problem is blood, lymph fluid, and gunk hanging around in the hole where the removed tissue resided. It takes a while for the body to reabsorb it.

From reading the posts in a chat room, I was pretty lucky. Some were so uncomfortable after lumpectomy they required constant medication to handle the pain. And it could go on for six months or longer. Heck, I just itched and twinged a bit.

Martha was going to be my driver for the PET scan. Rick wanted to be my chemotherapy babysitter. Rather than focusing on the scary big things, I whined that I didn't want a port stuck in my chest.

I had a needlepoint pillow to sew, two canvases of my own to finish, and Katie's Christmas presents to wrap, pack, and mail. Not to mention the desktop sitting in front of the couch and dusty furniture and dirty floors. Lunch. Could I have lunch?

The Port

Monday, December 5, 2011

You know how you can obsess over something? I was getting that way about the chest port, imagining this medical blob on my chest, hurting every time I moved, stopping me from taking baths. So I went back to the ever-obliging Internet.

The nurses need a catheter (a tube) to pour chemo drugs into your body. They could do it through an IV in your arm, but the drugs are nasty enough that they can mess up the IV and the delicate veins in your arm. Think of pouring acid through a straw into a plastic soda bottle. The acid will eat at the straw and it will eat at the soda bottle. Pour the acid a bunch of times; watch the straw and bottle spring leaks. You need a better method.

Replace the plastic bottle with a glass olive oil bottle with a rubber cork. Now, make a steel funnel with a tip small enough to go through the cork. Pour the acid through the funnel, through the cork, directly into the olive oil bottle. Voila! The steel and glass can withstand the acid so much better than plastic. You can pour acid through the funnel and into the bottle repeatedly without springing a leak.

The chest port is the olive oil bottle. Some have a rubber stopper on top (a needle is stuck through your skin and into the stopper) and some have a tube that sticks out of your skin (the drugs are poured through the tube.) The doctors know which type of port will work best for you. Users swear it makes chemotherapy sessions easier.

Peripherally inserted central catheters (PICC) go into a large vein near the elbow of the arm. Central line, tunneled venous catheters, or Hickman catheters, go into the chest by the collarbone or in the neck. Implantable ports or port-a-cath, can go in the arm or in the chest. Ports can stay put for months, even years.

It only hurts a little when they put it in. Depending on what kind they use, you will be given a topical anesthetic or be put to sleep while they thread the tubes and place the port.

The usual cautions about infection apply: keep things clean. If you show signs of infection, call the doctor. Other side effects are blood clots (characterized by soreness, swelling, or redness on the same side of the body as the port) and a blocked (clogged) line, which the nurse or doctor can determine. A port could shift, making it harder to get to or impossible to use. Worse comes to worse, they have to remove it.

Once the cut from putting the port in healed, I'd be able to take baths instead of showering.

I would have the implantable kind. Exactly how does it work? They buried the port just below my skin roughly midway between the middle of my breast and shoulder. As the drawing illustrates, when the nurse wanted to use it, she found the center by lightly pushing around it with her fingers. She then stuck a needle into the port. I got a prick through my skin, just like with any needle, but other than that, I didn't feel pain. To me, it hurt less than when they drew blood out of my arm.

A little knowledge goes a long way. I felt so much better!

This afternoon, I had an echocardiogram. It is a simple ultrasound test that bounces sound waves off the different parts of your heart. Very unthreatening, non-invasive, and fast. Then I went Christmas shopping. I'd had too much of the medical world. It was hard crawling into the real world, but I was going to practice.

Friday, December 9, 2011

This report was delayed; it was uncomfortable to type, so I didn't. Blame the chest port.

It sat high on the right side of my chest, below where Rick would pin a corsage, if I had a corsage and if I had him put it on the right side, which I didn't and I don't. And it wasn't as bad as imagination painted it.

How did it get in? That was Wednesday morning, running into the afternoon. Rick and I were at Henry Ford Hospital, this time at the Interventional Radiology Unit. Whatever the name means, they did pretty serious stuff there. I had to disrobe for one of those runway-ready gowns, keeping only my underwear. Bras are not underwear.

A pleasant male nurse took my blood pressure and verified that I hadn't eaten since the night before. Then a female nurse (darn, I enjoyed that guy fawning over me) tried to put an IV into the vein on the inside of my right forearm. The vein collapsed (the proper term, believe it or not, is that the vein blew.) Never had that happen before, but she explained the needle was probably too big for the vein. I didn't feel anything, but I did get a spectacular purple bruise there. So the IV went into my hand.

They let Rick in. That guy can go to Florida and run into someone he knows, so don't be surprised that he recognized a man in one of the other beds. They both work in the Renaissance Center in downtown Detroit. They chatted and then Rick kept vigil with me, waiting for the doctor. It took over an hour for someone to show up other than nurses asking, "Has the doctor come yet?" We didn't get an explanation or apology, but I think they had an emergency to tend before they could bother with me. Hindsight is 20/20: were they waiting for my soaring blood pressure to drop to a more reasonable level?

But then I had enough doctors to satisfy anyone. There were three; one of whom was definitely The Doctor. They had to explain the dangers of the procedure to me so I could sign an informed consent. The woman, thin and a little too brusque to suit me, was irritated when I told her it didn't matter what the risks were, I was having this done anyway.

I rolled my eyes at Rick, I think, and then I told them that the biggest risk was they could blow a hole through my artery or heart and I could die. The doctor agreed with me, but said they don't generally do things like that. Thank God for dry wit.

They shove the tube for the port through the vein until they nudge the heart, and then they back it off a bit. It can make the heart beat badly, but it is usually only one or two beats and then back to normal business. I wouldn't have a breathing tube—that was a whole other level of surgery. We got the formalities done.

I was wheeled down the hall and into the operating area, which was cluttered, but it wasn't the actual operating room.

There, I had a plethora of nice people introduce themselves and tell me what they were going to do. Most important at the moment was the girl who was going to feed me happy juice through the IV. Most people went to sleep, although some stayed awake, but I wouldn't feel any pain, just maybe some tugging and pushing. I told her I would snore.

A man held something to my neck. It was very cold and kind of burned, like a super-efficient ice cube. He was checking if I was "open" and I was. They put tape on my breast to simulate gravity as if I were standing. Then I was out. Two seconds of drifting and I was gone. And yes, I snored, because several times I heard myself snoring. I also knew that my throat was uber dry, so dry it ached. I wasn't conscious enough to try to swallow.

Anyway, when I woke up in my slot in the waiting room, the doctor had made a one inch slit in my chest, slid in a doodad, threaded the doodad's pipe into my vein, stitched me up on the inside, and painted plastic skin over the slit. I was now the proud possessor of a Vaccess CT power injectable port. Power injectable was good because the doctors could use that type to shoot me up with radioactive junk for MRIs and suchlike tests.

I foresaw lots of radioactive sessions in my future. I was pretty proud that I woke up rather quickly. Small things matter when you have no control.

They wanted my slot, so they shooed me and Rick into a room down the hall, me ensconced on my bed and he under power of feet. There we had to stay until 2:10 pm, just to make sure that my heart wasn't going to go spastic after the procedure. I got a bland basic sandwich, apple juice, yummy cookies, and an apple. Rick ate in the cafeteria while I snored.

It was now 2:25. We could leave. I needed to find Trish for an EKG. A wheelchair pusher had been ordered, but had not arrived. Hesitantly, the nurses decided Rick could get me to the 13th floor.

Trish really was cheerful, you know? She showed up, got me to a room, and got the technician. That girl stuck five or six little discs in various places on my front, hooked up the wires, and let me listen to my heart go pitter, pitter, pitter. No patters—it was as even as a metronome. The echocardiogram went as smooth as glass and so did the EKG. I had a solid, reliable heart.

My blood pressure was also reliable. I could rely on it going sky-high every time I had something done related to breast cancer. For the chest port procedure, the first blood pressure was 177 over whatever. They checked it several times; Rick said it was lower each time: 166 over something, then 143 over another number. Funny, no one asked if I had high blood pressure (hypertension,) which I did not.

Then, we could go home. Why, oh why, did every visit to this place turn into a full day? I was so glad to be outside, I didn't mind that it was cold. The valets were not rushing—it was obviously a full day of them taking cars and getting cars. Ours finally showed up and Rick poured me in.

We had to pick up Martha's jacket from the tailor and my coat from the dry cleaner. I waited in the car while Rick ran the errands. It was not my chest that was sore. It was my neck. Every little jerk from the movement of the car hurt where the guy had made it ice cold. I wanted to get home and sit. Vegetate. Make sure I was still alive.

Yes, I was alive. It was not so much pain as discomfort. Pressure in the chest: I had to get used to having a private needle holder under my skin. My vein had to calm down from a tube running through it (that was the pain in the neck.) My skin was scraped in two places, one of which roughly matched where the nurse checked if I was "open." (More reason for the pain in my neck. I have a small scar there.) That was the spot that bothered me the most.

Wednesday night, I slept upright in the chair because laying down flat was downright unpleasant. Last night I slept in the bed, though I felt a little weird. Tonight should be a breeze. But I shouldn't bend over and couldn't lift things. We had to get the port settled in my chest before I did acrobatics like driving a car. It needed seven to ten days of me being nice to my body, but I could shower. I was content to laze around. I had to take Benadryl to keep the plastic band-aid from itching to death.

Trish worked out my treatment calendar. I would have chemotherapy every three weeks. A lab was done every week. Labs were when they drew blood (I called them blood tests, not being a nurse,) checking to see if I was a walking time bomb ready to blow. No blood test, no chemo. That was the rule. I could have the tests done at Cottage Hospital, so the weekly visits would be as unobtrusive as possible. I thought the chest port would be a lifesaver; they could draw blood through that and save my hands and arms for silly things like typing and washing hair. (Wrong. No one was allowed to use the chest port except the chemotherapy people.)

There would be six chemo sessions. We would see if I could keep the schedule; they would have to postpone things if my blood counts got too wacky or if I was too sickly—if I couldn't stand the pace.

Monday, December 12, 2011

Off to Dr. Sanatio, this time for my sinuses. I had another infection. Oh, joy. It's a chronic headache and my biggest worry about chemotherapy. If chemo lowered my immunity, my sinuses could go into overdrive. Hope my head didn't fall off.

I stopped at Cottage Hospital and learned that I did not need appointments to have blood work done. Just show up during their extended office hours and show them the authorization slip.

Katie wanted to come in February to help. She had maxed out her vacation time—use it or lose it—and I think she felt helpless in Sacramento while I was in Detroit suffering. She would rent a car and ferry me to and from chemo—do whatever needed doing, take care of me. Sure, we'd be delighted to have her anytime. I hoped I was not too sickly to enjoy her presence.

Wednesday, December 14, 2011

The hardest part of a PET scan is the diet one must follow beforehand, and that was not incredibly difficult. Take up the Atkins diet for a day—all protein, no sugar, no carbs—and you have the PET scan diet licked. Then, don't have anything but water for six hours before the appointment. It was as easy as pie, but I sure would have liked a slice. Blueberry, please. The reason for the diet was that they shoot radioactive sugar into your veins, which glows anywhere there is metabolic activity and shows up on the scan. I guess cancer cells are famous for their metabolic activity. The diet is so you have as little sugar as possible floating around, causing metabolic activity. Protein makes the least sugar.

They had me take a Xanax one hour before the appointment. Something about the pill relaxes your innards as well as your mind and the PET scan can see into your body easier. Something about the relaxation made it a heck of a lot easier for me to go through the scanner. Remember the trouble I had with the MRI? Didn't notice the PET scanner swallowing me.

I drank well-watered, lemon flavored radioactive gunk. They IV'ed more gunk into my arm (no, they didn't use my chest port. They were not authorized to do so.) I could feel it run through me as warmth. Then I sat and studied my fingernails for an hour while the glow in the dark effect got into all my nooks and crannies. Then into the scanner. Done!

Everything in life could go back to normal. Drink lots of fluids for a couple of days to flush the radioactivity out. But don't bother going to the airport. I would set off the scanners and they would drag me into a room, interrogate me, strip search me. Maybe ship me off to Gitmo and waterboard me. Waterboarding would help flush the radioactivity out. (And pull myself together! What a thing to joke about. Gitmo indeed.)

The results of the PET scan would be available Friday. I'd see if Trish could check it for me. The plastic skin around the chest port incision was just beginning to pull loose at the edges. And my sinuses felt loads better, thanks to antibiotics.

Friday, December 16, 2011

Trish called yesterday. It turned out I was not eligible for the clinical study after all—it was for Tc3 tumors and I was Tc1—Stage III versus Stage I—but she had another I might be able to participate in. So, I took Martha to work and then ran up the freeway to Henry Ford Hospital.

Trish and I went through the second clinical trial plans and I signed the papers. The second study did not interest me nearly as much as the first; there wasn't any direct benefit in fighting the cancer, but I would receive a drug that might help keep my white blood cell (WBC) count up. That stuff fights infections and with my sinuses, well, I might need all the help I could get. I had to pee into a cup to check for kidney trouble.

The most upsetting part was that Trish postponed my first chemotherapy session, probably for a week, while we straightened out the clinical studies. I didn't want it postponed, but was obedient. Good little girl, Ann, have some ice cream. It'll make you feel better.

Trish copied the reports I had not already received, including the one from the PET scan. From them I learned the reason they harvested two lymph nodes during my lumpectomy rather than one: on the operating table, they injected radioactive blue dye into my breast and waited a few minutes. One lymph node turned blue, so they grabbed that one. But there seemed to still be radioactivity hanging around, so they pulled the second lymph node out. That one wasn't blue.

What they dug out with the ice cream scoop: it went from the chest wall out toward my nipple. The two bits mentioned in the pathology report that Dr. Medica was going to ask about? No firm answer, but Trish told me that it's not uncommon. They probably weren't cancer, just little spots. Not to worry. No sign of a pathology report, but the DCIS was the same as the invasive tumor: triple negative.

Now the results of the PET scan, some parts in the language fondly known as Gobbledygook:

I had an impressive list of normal limits. In the neck, my maxillary sinuses and thyroid gland were fine. No cervical lymphadenopathy and the airways were patent. Down further, the liver looked happy, as did the gallbladder, pancreas, spleen, adrenal glands, kidneys, and the stomach. The small bowel and colon were ready to go.

I did have several uninflamed sigmoid diverticula, which is common enough. It can become diverticulitis. We should all eat more fiber, then maybe we wouldn't develop those pouches. Also, my abdominal aorta was minimally calcified without complications. Oops, sounds like something to discuss with Dr. Sanatio. He'd probably tell me to clamp down more on cholesterol. Yes, sir, will do. Cancel that order for ice cream.

We should throw computers and TVs out the window. Live on farms, get our exercise pulling weeds, live off the land instead of the overly processed food we get from grocery store freezers. We would be healthier. Then again, we'd get more skin cancer from all that time in the great outdoors, right? I heard that they tested a bunch of Egyptian mummies and found that about half of them had evidence of heart disease. Sounds like a design flaw God never got around to fixing.

In the chest, there were no enlarged supraclavicular, mediastinal, or hilar lymph nodes. Since they were ok, who cares what they are? One lymph node on the left side was mildly prominent with slightly thickened cortex and mild degree of FDG uptake. The FDG uptake was the drug glowing, but it was more likely that the lymph node was doing its work fighting infection (take that, sinuses) than that it was dealing with metastatic cancer.

There was an area in my left breast that didn't look so good, which "might represent either post-biopsy reactive changes or residual malignancy." We would get the chemotherapy done and then check again, Trish assured me. But there was "no evidence of the osseous or solid organs metastasis." I didn't know the technical words, but I could read the sentence fine. No evidence of metastasis. The cancer had not spread.

PET scans are extraordinary things.

I took myself home and sat down to read the papers for the second clinical study. It was a Phase III clinical trial comparing the combination of TC (my chemo drugs) plus Bevacizumab (the drug they were testing) to TC alone and to TAC (another combination of chemo drugs) for women with node-positive or high risk node negative (me) Her-2/neu negative (me) breast cancer. In plain English, they wanted to find out of if Bevacizumab helps other drugs fight cancer more than they already know it does.

The list of side effects would give Yoda pause. The common ones sounded about the same as the list for the first study. The "Less likely—occur in 3-9%"—included such nasty things as intestinal blockage, blood clots, and heart failure. It was the "Rare but serious" side effects that scared the liver out of me. If my liver stayed in my body, it could fail. Heart attack and heart failure, lung damage that could be permanent, perforation of the stomach or bowel, kidney failure, blood clots, tissue death, acute leukemia; these were all side effects.

What had I gotten myself into? I turned on the computer.

The drug being tested was Bevacizumab. It was used to treat other types of cancers. Now they were trying to figure out if it was effective against breast cancer. BUT...

The FDA decided Bevacizumab was not sufficiently effective treating women with Stage IV breast cancer to approve its use for breast cancer treatment. It didn't work well enough for women who were dying of breast cancer to make them ignore the horrible side effects. So what makes them think it would help me, measly little Stage I cancer fighter that I was? I was not in imminent danger of dying. But if I did the study and took Bevacizumab, I upped my risk of croaking.

I called Trish to tell her I was not going to do the second study. I talked to her answering machine. A while later, I called the main line and asked if I was still scheduled for chemotherapy Monday. No, but Trish could put me back on the list.

I gave up and called her again to tell her I was going to have my blood drawn at Cottage Hospital; if I didn't get the blood test done, I couldn't have chemo Monday no matter what.

I would like to start chemo on Monday!

After I got back from Cottage, there was a message on my answering machine. No, I would not start chemo Monday, but Trish would call me.

Then I emailed Katie and told her not to get a plane ticket yet. The February date for my chemotherapy might change. And I stopped taking the antibiotic for my sinuses. I didn't know if it would clash with the chemo drugs and figured safe was better than sorry.

Chemotherapy Cycle 1

Suggested Shopping List

- Comfortable clothing that will give access to a chest port (opens in front and/or can be easily pulled down or pushed aside—and I do mean easily. It has to stay out of the way for hours.) and bares upper arm for blood pressure cuffs. For an example, look at my picture in the back of the book. I am wearing one of my chemo shirts
- Something to do while sitting quietly for two or more hours—books, magazines, Kindle, IPad, etc. (don't count on Internet access.) You could knit, etc., provided swinging your arm doesn't disturb the IV
- Gallons of bottled water to drink (not carbonated.) If your area has high quality tap water, you might not need bottled water, but you do need gallons
- A bottle or two of expensive Perrier water to mix with regular water for taste (optional)
- High protein foods: prepackaged meats, cheese, and other foods—nothing from a deli—no caffeine or carbonation—no fresh vegetables (frozen is okay)—choose a bland diet until you know what your stomach will tolerate. Think comfort food for a sore mouth and unhappy stomach but concentrate on protein and a balanced diet
- Fruit juice (possibly only low acid)
- Thick skinned fruits like oranges and bananas
- High quality chapstick
- Heartburn medication (Tums or similar) just in case
- Cottonelle wipes or similar (optional)
- Non-alcoholic mouthwash
- Mild toothpaste with fluoride
- High quality multivitamin

- B-Complex vitamins (even though the multivitamin has B in it)
- Medical face masks (for protection from other people's germs) (optional)
- Refresh eye drops or similar (not Visine)
- High quality/high powered skin lotion
- Ibuprofen (not aspirin or Tylenol. Only Ibuprofen has anti-inflammatory properties that are beneficial)
- Ocean (saline spray for the nose) (optional)
- Biotine for the mouth (optional)
- Preparation H cream, not suppositories (optional)
- Antibacterial soap to wash fruits, countertops, etc.
- Kotex or similar—absolutely no tampons (if you have periods)
- A hat, scarf, turban or wig
  Yes, I know some of it sounds silly or excessive, but read on.

Monday, December 19, 2011

Trish called. No, I couldn't do the first clinical trial, and no, I didn't want to do the second. But I could start chemotherapy tomorrow, if I didn't want to wait until after Christmas. No! My emotions said Christmas was not as important as staying alive.

Okay, be at Henry Ford Hospital at 8 am. Goody, I didn't waste a blood test. Sadly, Trish would no longer be my personal assistant. She was secretary for clinical trial patients only. After dinner, I got up my courage and peeled the plastic skin off the chest port incision. It was looser than I thought and came off pretty easily.

To keep myself occupied, I did more research. There are support groups out there. I didn't contact any, other than the one phone call to the American Cancer Society back in November. But I am an introverted loner; the typical writer. I'd be happy on a desert island with just my Man Friday to keep me company. If I needed to bitch or complain, I had a husband and two daughters to listen. I got information off the Internet or from Henry Ford. Heck, I was writing this as my chosen form of therapy. You might want or need more.

Start with the American Cancer Society. They have a web site; they have phones. They can steer you to whatever support is available, whether it's a group meeting in a church, restaurant or hospital. If you need help dealing with feelings, find a therapist—someone to talk to who can provide competent guidance. If you feel stymied, ask your doctor for suggestions or a referral.

There is lots of help out there. Get it, as much as you need. Fighting cancer is complex, both physically and mentally. Arm yourself with all the weapons you can use. Rah, team, fight.

Tuesday, December 20, 2011

Today was the first chemo treatment AKA Cycle 1. I tend to be OCD about being on time for appointments, so I was a little tenser than I would have been if everyone had gotten up good this morning. As it was, both Rick and Martha dragged their feet. We got to the hospital with five minutes to spare; signed in and sat down. Hurry up and wait. I was called in half an hour later.

Weighed, blood pressure and temperature tested, we were ushered into a huge room. It was a big U with locked doors at both ends so you can't just wander in, bathrooms and a nurse's office, and maybe a closet or three in the center, and lines of Lazy Boys and equipment going around. Desks at the bottom of the U were for the staff.

In a small room at one curve of the U, a nurse scrubbed at the skin around my chest port and then stuck the IV apparatus into the port. The apparatus was a sideways needle that stuck into the chest port through the skin. Attached to the needle was a long IV line (a tube) with two more lines branching from it, so they could give me two shots of whatever at once. The whole was covered with a large clear plastic bandage that kept everything in place and covered the port for cleanliness, leaving the IV lines hanging outside where they could be reached. Having the needle go in pricked, but actually was less bothersome than a regular IV or a shot. If I wanted, I could get a prescription for a cream that deadens the feeling.

The nurse praised my shirt—I bought two from Roaman's catalog just for chemo. Short sleeves, so there was full access to my arm for blood pressure cuffs, scoop-necked and full button down the front, giving good access to the chest port. Once the IV was set up, I saw an additional benefit to the shirt. The material was gauzy cotton, not great for winter wear, but light enough that the material did not pull on the chest port stuff. They were busy prints, kind of African in nature, so I could go braless and still be modest (bra straps cut across the chest port and felt weird) a little oversize, so very comfy. Not the highest quality but they were good for doctor's visits and chemo. Once this was all done, I would throw them away. I had a cardigan in case I got cold.

Sherry was nurse for the day. She ushered me to my decadent couch. Actually, I was to sit on a generic Naugahyde Lazy Boy with attached trays, on one either side. An IV stand with an automatic control box stood to the side. There was a chair for Rick, not nearly as comfortable as my Lazy Boy. A pillow and blankets waited, but I was hot. I shouldn't wear sweat pants. It may be cold out, but it was a lot warmer in the hospital than in my house.

With our stuff stashed at our station, Sherry gave us the grand tour. There were four bathrooms, two on each side of the U, and a little refrigerator stocked with apple juice and snacks. Rather basic, but much better than nothing. There were a few other people in Lazy Boys, but not many. The ones who were there frankly didn't look very healthy.

This was training day as well as chemo day. Sherry hooked me up to the IV and started a saline drip. Drip that water in, hydrate me so the drugs worked well. Rick and I watched a video on cancer that was soothing, although I could have guessed or already knew most of the info in it. During it, I ate the crackers I brought from home and washed them down with water. They were an adequate, if not great, breakfast, and had the added benefit of not being hard on my stomach, which was frog jumping. Then the video was done and Sherry returned.

The information came hard and fast. First, if someone had an emergency, they would be surrounded by nurses who knew exactly what to do, so don't panic. I was Stage I and she had every faith that I would have a good outcome, but that was not true of many of the people receiving chemo today. Plenty of them were staving off death as best they may.

Sherry filled us in on the schedule and procedures. Normally, one sees the doctor the day before chemo, but since all my appointments had already been scheduled by Trish, we would not upset the apple cart and change things. Chemo weeks, I would come in Tuesdays at 9 am, see the doctor and have my blood drawn, and then have the chemo treatment at 11. The weeks I didn't have chemo, I must have my blood drawn at Cottage Hospital. Do it every Tuesday, no exceptions, no excuses. No bloodwork, no chemo. The doctor reviewed the blood work; if anything was off, it was dealt with. Don't be surprised if I got a phone call at 2 am—the doctor had been known to do that if she was sufficiently alarmed by blood counts.

The schedule is all-important. The sessions are timed to catch and kill cancer cells. A disruption gives random cells to a chance to slip through the net. So, hope the doctors don't decide there has to be a rest period at some point. The gap isn't ideal for killing cancer, and also indicates you are not responding very well to treatment in some way.

Sherry had a copy of my latest blood test and went over it with us. What counted most were the Hemoglobin and Neutrophil counts. They were added together; as long as the total was over 1200, I was in good shape. If they dropped below 1200 but were still above 500, my immune system was not happy, but I did have some ability to fight infection. If they dropped below 500, warning bells went off and chances were chemotherapy would be postponed.

What could I do to help? Eat well. Lots of protein—if I couldn't do protein, do the best I could. A high quality (not a cheapie) full spectrum vitamin was essential, especially during chemo, when eating a well-balanced diet was a challenge. Centrum Chewables were a great choice.

Avoid sources of infection. Sources of infection were more than just staying out of crowds. The least obvious were foods. Thick skinned fruit like bananas and oranges were okay. Stay away from fresh veggies and forget thin skinned fruit like strawberries. Frozen vegetables worked. Don't get anything from a deli— no sliced cheese unless it was prepackaged from the manufacturer—nothing that had been allowed to sit out anywhere. Eat potato salad and die. Anything fresh that had skin should be rinsed well, perhaps washed with a drop of antibiotic soap. I jokingly suggested that Stouffers and Lean Cuisines were my best bet, and Sherry agreed. If it was pre-prepared, prepackaged, homogenized, and I handled it carefully, it would be okay.

Don't eat anything a fly landed on—flies are dirty, dirty, dirty. Bacteria is everywhere, and if my immune system was suppressed, it could take me down. Eating it was asking for serious trouble.

Wash kitchen counters as if there was no tomorrow. Wash my hands a lot. Watch out for cuts on the skin—a hangnail or paper cut needed careful care. Keep track of the anus (ugh, not a topic most people care to get into) because hemorrhoids and little cracks from constipation can get infected. Irritation from the runs is nearly as dangerous. A face mask can't hurt—I saw enough of them at Henry Ford Hospital to guess they were the newest fad.

Drink lots of liquids—dehydration was to be avoided at all costs. Two to three quarts of liquid a day if I could. If I did get dehydrated, they would haul me in and get the water level up by IV. It was important to
- Flush the drugs throughout my body
- Flush the drugs out of my body

Side effects get in the way.

Sherry moved on to how the IV's were handled—the dosage was by my weight; I got two drugs, Taxotere and Cytoxan. They were not administered at the same time, but one after another. I wasn't chained to the chair, just to the IV. The IV controller had a battery so it could be unplugged from the wall so I could go to the bathroom and kitchen. To recline the chair, just push back on the head. I tried it, but preferred to sit upright.

There would be prescriptions to fill; would I like to use the hospital pharmacy, in which case they were delivered to me on my Lazy Boy throne, or would I prefer to have them filled elsewhere? Without thinking, I agreed to get them there.

The doctor signed off on my treatment. We had liftoff. Sherry hooked up the Taxotere and kept busy by setting up the shot to give me if I had an allergic reaction to the drug. She didn't just get the stuff out, she got a hypodermic needle loaded and ready. Better safe than sorry. She filled me in on the symptoms to watch for, and watched me to make sure I didn't blossom with anything suspicious. It was twenty minutes of watching. I didn't have any symptoms, so we could relax.

Sherry turned the IV speed up to normal so I got the drug quicker. She could turn it up a little faster, but it tended to make the sinuses burn a little. No, I didn't need to upset my sinuses.

Rick and I came prepared with books. I had brought a good book to focus my attention. Still, I had trouble keeping my eyes on the page. I only interrupted myself once to go to the bathroom before the hour of Taxotere was up. I sipped water and apple juice. My crackers were done. Rick escaped for a coffee run; he can't live without coffee.

When the buzzer on the IV controller went off, Sherry hooked up the Cytoxan. It doesn't like plastic, so it was in a different bag with different IV lines. This drug would take an hour and a half to trickle into me. We should be out at 1:15.

I didn't feel anything with the Taxotere, but the Cytoxan gradually painted a metallic taste in my mouth. It wasn't extreme, but when Rick fetched me some orange juice, it didn't taste right. I went back to water. Then I burped. My stomach was a little distended; I had gas. Other than burping once in a while, going to the bathroom again and suffering a funky aftertaste in my mouth, I was fine.

When the Cytoxan was done, Sherry did a flush (shooting liquid in with a hypodermic needle) of the chest port with heparin to facilitate clotting and unhooked me. The pharmacy had not delivered my prescriptions so she called them. Because it was our first time, they needed insurance information. We went downstairs to the pharmacy, slowly dealt with the overworked staff, and got three prescriptions.

- Decadron AKA Dexamethasone—I was to take this corticosteroid before and after every chemo treatment. It helps with inflammation and immune stimulation.
- Prochlorperazine—60 tablets. Anti-nausea drug. Take every six

hours as needed. It amused me that this drug was used to treat nausea, schizophrenia and generalized nonpsychotic anxiety. Guess which diagnosis applied to me? No, you only think anxiety counted.

- Ondansetron—12 tablets. This was the Superman of anti-nausea drugs. If I was going somewhere and must not throw up, take this. They don't give many because the insurance companies don't want to pay for it.

Obviously, they expected me to get nauseated. Chemo does that. It's probably it's most famous side effect.

Anti-nausea drugs are a boon, but can also be a bust. They cause side effects, folks. Prochlorperazine can make you dizzy, jittery, or give you muscle spasms. That's not a complete list; it can get nasty. Others can bring you down with dry mouth, stuffy nose, coordination problems, fatigue, diarrhea, headaches, blurred vision, constipation, and abdominal pain. Don't hesitate to take the drugs if you need them, but it might be a balancing act between settling your stomach and other hazards.

Maybe they figured I was going to be nauseated, but I was not. I was hungry. We ended up at Nathan's Deli scarfing down sandwiches and pop (soda to the world outside the Midwest.) I only drank a quarter of the can because I was burping and didn't really want the carbonation. With the drug taste in my mouth, the only thing that tasted exactly as it should was chocolate. God's gift to mankind! (Was the biblical manna chocolate?)

I blew my nose. Eewww. Bright yellow snot. That brought it home that these drugs really go throughout the body. Before I went to sleep, I put Refresh eye drops in. They were supposed to flush the drugs out of my eyes—the drugs can mess with the tear ducts, even narrow them, and it takes surgery to fix it. Do the eye drops religiously several times a day for three days, minimum.

Really, if I didn't know what I did all day, it would have been a normal night.

Wednesday, December 21, 2011

The bad taste in my mouth receded until it was hardly noticeable. I felt a bit shaky; but nothing else. I pretty much felt normal, even energetic. And relieved. The wait, wait, wait was done.

Side effects vary from person to person with no guess to what I would be hit with. They generally show up three days after chemo, although some people don't get them until five days into the cycle. Neilu, a girl Katie worked with, started side effects ten days after her chemo treatments, but she had a different type of cancer. I was curious as to what I would suffer.

I was a good girl and took the Decadron on schedule. I used eye drops twice during the day and again before I went to bed.

Thursday, December 22, 2011

I had diarrhea every time I went to the bathroom. Not bad diarrhea, but not firm stools. After a couple of days of that, my rear end hurt.

Trouble coming. My ears were ringing and my sinuses were acting up. I should call the doctor and find out what they wanted me to do—tomorrow was my last chance until Tuesday, probably, to see someone outside the emergency room. Joyeux Noël. (Didn't manage to do it.)

I peed more than I took in. That's a no no. Gulped water all afternoon to avoid getting dehydrated. I am a sipper, not a gulper.

I looked up a side effect. If you have not gone through menopause, you can experience irregular vaginal bleeding, dribs or drabs, during chemo. It might be your period, but report it to the doctor anyway. It may be that it isn't your period at all, but bleeding caused by a blood clotting problem or other imbalance of blood levels. Lord knows the blood gets messed up by chemo—you don't want it to get worse.

If you have gone through menopause and experience vaginal bleeding during chemo, you haven't gotten younger. You need to contact the doctor.

For both non and menopausal women, don't use tampons during chemo. You are at higher risk of infection, and tampons are a way to introduce infection-causing agents into your body.

Thanks to lowered blood estrogen, vaginal dryness is a common side effect of chemo. This can make intercourse painful or impossible. Liberal use of water based lubricants such as K-Y jelly, Lubrin, Surgilube or Astroglide for sexual activity may solve the problem. If they don't, speak to the doctor. There are other products available but a prescription may be required. (K-Y jelly may be the slipperiest thing in the world. A kitten got its head stuck in the fancy spokes of a car tire's wheel cover. They tried all sorts of stuff to help slide it out without success. One messy kitten later, K-Y jelly did the trick.)

My hair was going to fall out. For a woman who turned her nose up at narcissism, it was disheartening to realize how much I dreaded losing it. I liked my hair just the way it was, not long, maybe six inches from scalp to non-split ends. Regardless, I had nightmares of waking up with detached hair coating my pillow, clogging my mouth, nose and ears. It'd be all over the furniture and floor. That would be gross.

I handed Martha a pair of scissors and told her to cut it short. She took me at my word and I turned into Mia Farrow, with one inch long hair all over my head. Going slowly in deference to my tingling, weird feeling scalp, Martha did a decent job of it.

Taxotere can cause folliculitis, as in a really itchy scalp. The follicles (where the hair comes from) become inflamed. At first it may look like small red bumps or white-headed pimples. You shouldn't ignore it because it can spread and get nasty. (I had a touch of it—that is why my head felt strange.)

One lady had folliculitis—it looked like diaper rash on her head to her—and she found advice on the Internet. Wash her head with Dial soap and put hydrogen peroxide on the bumps. Her comment?

"So you are bald and blond or is it blond and bald?"

Love her sense of humor but forget the harsh stuff. Doctors say to use baby shampoo on your head, Eucerin on the rash, take Benadryl for the itch, and sleep in a skull cap.

Friday, December 23, 2011

My mouth was sore—I had a few white streaks on the side of my tongue. It was mucositis, inflammation and thinning of the mucous membranes. Mucous membranes are fast growing cells. This makes them look like cancer to the chemo drugs, which are designed to seek out the speedy, but are not smart enough to tell the difference between good and evil. The Taxotere and Cytoxan were overdoing their job and breaking down the mucous membranes in my mouth.

Mucositis can turn into painful sores, bleeding and infection. The full symptoms are dryness and burning of the lips and mouth, patches on the tongue, inside the mouth, and down the throat, vaginal and rectal itching, burning, redness, sores or dryness, a feeling of having a lump in your throat, swelling, and difficulty swallowing. (I confused it with thrush.)

It was just in my mouth; the upshot was that it didn't feel good to eat. I skipped garlic toast and just ate spaghetti. The ice cream I had for dessert was soothing, and because it was chocolate, it tasted good. Nothing tasted good except chocolate. I preferred drinks lukewarm, although my brain said "ick" to non-iced water. I rinsed my mouth out with salt water and that eased it temporarily.

The upside was that mucous membranes regenerate quickly, so the mucositis should be limited time-wise. Still, I called the Breast Cancer clinic and they arranged for a prescription of "magic mouthwash" to ease the symptoms. It was not an immediate fix.

If this was the extent of my side effects, I would survive.

Monday, December 26, 2011

Arrogance bites you in the butt every time. Yes, I would survive, but now I understood how for some people the cure is worse than the illness. Let us run through Christmas, shall we?

Magic mouthwash was a combination of Nystatin, Benadryl, and Lidocaine. It numbs your mouth—if you are desperate and swallow it, it also numbs the part of your throat that hurts. One teaspoon four times a day and you can talk around the soreness of your tongue rubbing against your teeth. Tongues don't hurt against teeth, you say? With mucositis they can. But with magic mouthwash you can eat. You can also sleep, which isn't the easiest thing to do when your mouth hurts.

So I got my magic mouthwash, ate dinner and watched TV. It might be my imagination, but the magic mouthwash restored taste buds a trifle. Not much, but enough so I could taste something other than dirt.

Iron Chef America was on at 11 pm. I usually watch it and then go to bed. Friday night I watched about 10 minutes. Then I was in the bathroom for more than 45 minutes, just sitting on the toilet in a cold sweat, hanging onto the window sill and sink, thinking I might fall asleep, pass out, or melt into the toilet. I'm not sure what it was, if the chemicals had dug deep, or what, but I felt dreadful. Absolutely like I was going to die.

The worst was that I forgot why I was doing this to myself. Cancer was the furthest thing from my mind. I decided that I would not go through this again. I had a bit of the runs, but not enough to make a difference, and no cramps. The cold sweat was its own symptom, independent of anything else.

My face was gray and my skin looked pockmarked, rough, like all the pores opened wide and stayed open. I finally pried myself off the toilet and went to bed. My ears were pounding and though it's not a good idea to self-medicate, I took an antibiotic. I had four; they would get me through till Tuesday when I could reach the doctor. I hoped.

The cold sweat dried up, I warmed up, and fell asleep.

I slept two hours, then I was up for four. Not that I felt that bad, I just didn't feel good. When I woke, I had a vague feeling of panic, as if my body knew it had poison in it that had to be expelled. The feeling was not strong; I overcame it easily, but I had to eat—had to drink something—then I had to wait for my system to realize it had gotten some fuel. Four hours, then I fell asleep for three or four hours.

When I woke, my tongue was coated. A thick white, unpalatable feeling and tasting coating covered my tongue. I thought it was thrush, a yeast (fungal) infection. I went to the Internet and found that Nystatin is an anti-fungal drug which works against thrush, and there was Nystatin in my magic mouthwash. Salvation was at hand. I swished, brushed my teeth and tongue as well as I could, and tried to eat. My mouth really stung. The chocolate ice cream Rick served me had bits of solid chocolate in it; I couldn't eat the bits. It was like sucking on walnuts.

Around 11 am, I began to feel better. Not good, but better. I was no longer a limp piece of decayed spaghetti propped up in a chair. I remembered to use the eye drops, swish my mouth, take a bath. Eat. Breathe. Live.

My daughter ran errands; an array of necessities for me at the top of her list. I told her what I needed and wanted, croaking like a frog because somewhere along the line, I got laryngitis. My throat didn't hurt, but I couldn't talk well. Using a flashlight, I admired the little boxing thing at the back of my mouth. It was bright red, matching the rest of my throat.

What I needed to survive:

- Wipes for my sore, bleeding anus. Persistent diarrhea had brought me low. My butt hurt and I bled every time I went to the bathroom. Cottonelle wipes felt very good.
- Fruit juice. Ginger ale and orange soda pop did not taste good. Sugar was cloying, bubbles felt nasty. I didn't try Coke or Pepsi because caffeine isn't recommended. Water was worse. Detroit's water is high quality—among the best in the nation. I liked the way it tasted. I just didn't like it with meals. From being an occasional sipper, I progressed to lusting after an ice-filled glass of water, one that tasted as it should. Thanks to chemo, it didn't taste good at all. Apple cranberry fruit juice tasted okayish, but I could feel acid in my mouth and against my lips. Good old purple grape juice, which normally I am not fond of, became my staple drink. Mixed with less water, it was a drink. Mixed with more water, it made drinkable water.
- Potatoes and bananas. Baked potatoes with lots of butter tasted okay. Bananas are good for you.

That was all I needed. I wasn't doing very well in the food department, was I? No, that wasn't all I ate. It was all I wanted.

I should have also wanted super-strength Blistex to coat my lips against the acid surging up my throat into my mouth (which I did not recognize as acid. That was what made my boxing bag red and made me lose my voice,) but I didn't think of it.

Martha also got pre-packaged deli meats and cheese, the kind packaged at the factory. They said that those should be sufficiently germ-free to eat. Remember, chemo lowers your immunity. It can get so bad, that the germs you usually eat safely can jump your bones and beat you to a pulp. Anything that sits out at a deli or restaurant—anything that is sliced on the slicer in the store—anything that isn't hermetically sealed at a factory isn't good.

If my immunity dropped to the bottom, the hospital would give me a shot of Neulasta. (I never got one, not once, through six chemotherapy cycles.) It is one of those wonder drugs; it boosts the immune system. It is in a class of medications called colony stimulating factors. It works by stimulating bone marrow to make more neutrophils, a type of blood cell needed to fight infection. The benefit of Neulasta, other than increasing immunity, is it strengthens the intensity of the chemo drugs. They give it to you the day after your chemo session. It may leave a lump or swelling that doesn't go away. If that happens, you are supposed to tell the doctor about it. Like many shots, it can also hurt for a while.

The serious side effects of Neulasta are:
- Rupture of the spleen, which can kill you. The spleen is located in the top left of your stomach. If you get a shot, and that area hurts, call the doctor right away. Your spleen might be enlarging, getting ready to explode.
- Acute respiratory distress syndrome. If you have trouble breathing after getting the shot, call the doctor or go to the emergency room.
- Serious allergic reactions. The reaction can happen while you are getting the shot or sometime after. Don't neglect it! Call the doctor or go to the emergency room.
- If you have Sickle Cell Anemia, tell the doctor before you get the shot. Neulasta can cause serious Sickle Cell crises. These are characterized by pain and breathing difficulty.

Neulasta can also bring on side effects:
- Vomiting
- Weakness
- Swelling of arms, hands, feet, ankles, or legs
- Headache
- Constipation
- Bone or muscle pain

Doesn't everything involved with chemotherapy do the same?

Back to Christmas Eve. Rick cooked a prime rib roast (one of his Christmas presents) and the oven smoked. No, I am not going to explain how I got a grease slick in the bottom of my oven, but I hadn't been aware it was bad enough to smoke up the house. Rick opened the kitchen window and front door to air the house out. The smoke made me feel sickly. Then he and Martha left for the Christmas Eve service at church.

I in my wisdom decided to clean the self-cleaning oven. Bad move. The smoke was thicker and I couldn't tolerate it. I switched off the oven and opened doors and windows again. Finally, I retreated to the bedroom with my heart pounding and some difficulty breathing. I think the lesson here is that chemotherapy reduces you to a hopeless, ailing lump. Things that your normal body can take will lay you low. I couldn't breathe right.

I slept two hours, woke up for four, and managed to get back to sleep. I woke at 10 am Christmas Day, starting to feel human. My tongue was not quite so coated; swish magic mouthwash every four hours without fail to thwart mucositis.

I was alert enough to open presents. I cried when Martha gave me a Kindle—it was to keep me occupied during chemo sessions. Later, I pulled my brain together enough to download True Blood, the HBO series based on the Sookie Stackhouse books. I like the books—hopefully I would enjoy the series enough to forget about what was happening in the chemo room. I cried when I figured out how to download the videos to the Kindle.

My brother called later and I cried again. Shall we say my emotions were close to the surface?

So were zits. My face broke out. I had pimples where I never had pimples on my face. I scratched one and it bled. I had to press Kleenex over it for five minutes to stop the bleeding. The coating on my tongue was down a little; I kept swigging mouthwash.

Hip hip hooray, Swiss cheese actually tasted like Swiss cheese. I ate four slices in celebration and regretted it. The fourth slice was one too many. I didn't get nauseated, but I felt a little queasy.

I did not want complicated food. Meat and cheese, applesauce, chocolate ice cream without anything in it. I had no desire for a sandwich, but I allowed Rick to feed me one, hoping the bulk would stop the runs. It didn't.

Call me Scrooge. I couldn't generate any Christmas cheer. The house still smelled like smoke and it made me feel yucky. I took a nap while Rick aired the house out again. After lolling around all day and night, I went to bed and actually slept 4 hours before I woke up. I was up for 2 hours and then back to sleep. Maybe I was coming out of it.

I was lucky, missing out on nausea, but the side effects I did suffer were as much as I could tolerate. I was not sure what future chemo sessions would bring—if I would stick to the same side effects, or add to them —but I was going to demand a stronger prescription to deal with my mouth.

I was not having difficulty swallowing, but did have trouble keeping my throat clear. Rather than having a dry mouth, as the side effect lists say will happen, I was making huge amounts of saliva; buckets of it filled my mouth and then, when I swallowed, it didn't want to go down easily. If I didn't pay attention when I swallowed, I choked. This was a bigger problem when I was trying to get to sleep.

Also, congestion associated with my sinuses—post nasal drip, drip, drip—was harder to clear. My throat was a little sore, whether from mucositis or infection or something else I couldn't tell. The result was I hacked my way through the day and night.

My intestines were not happy. Too much diarrhea for too long and I was now getting very vague cramps at times. I had been warned; chemo can make the stool go through your system faster, resulting in diarrhea, or slower, causing constipation. Yes, you can get cramps, also gas. If you have sudden severe pain, speed dial the doctor or go to the emergency room in case you have gotten a hole somewhere down there, as in perforation. Perforation of the bowel, for example, is a red alert emergency. Imagine smearing stool from your bowel into your stomach and you can understand the panic. Perforation kills.

To ease cramps, try lying down for a while or imagine yourself somewhere pleasant. Relax and breathe deeply.

I wanted to eat healthy, but there were obstacles to doing so, the most prominent being taste. I was doing the best I could. Martha went for pizza and it almost tasted normal, but way too spicy. My tongue was not precisely sore, but it was sensitive.

I had vague pains in the muscles in my thighs. My scalp itched. Not a normal itch, a duller itch. I could feel pimples on my scalp and the skin felt tight. I bet this was the beginning of losing my hair. I had Martha take a picture of my face to make a template of my eyebrows. Then, if they fell off, I could paint on realistic eyebrows. Hindsight is 20/20: I never painted on eyebrows. Didn't think of doing it. My looks were the least of my worries.

I had been taking the antibiotic and it kept my head from falling off, but my ears were ringing enough to play the finale of the 1812 Overture, complete with Civil War cannon. Guess what? Chemo can make your ears ring. The ringing is called tinnitus and is often associated with dizziness and nausea. It is a symptom of nerve damage, and turns out to be quite common. As to whether it was temporary or permanent, only time would tell. Checking in chat rooms, some lost the tinnitus and others didn't when they finished treatment.

Sound Pharmaceuticals, Inc., a biopharmaceutical company in Seattle, Washington, is working to develop drugs to help prevent hearing loss during chemotherapy. They are now (2012) conducting a study to test a drug which might help prevent damage, but the chemo drugs they consider most damaging were not the ones I received.

Sound Pharmaceuticals' explanation is:

There are three major groups of nerves in the human body.
- The peripheral nerves that carry information to and from the limbs.
- The nerves that supply the bowels and other internal organs.
- The nerves of the head which connect to ears, eyes, taste buds, etc.

Nerves in any or all of these major groups can be affected by certain chemotherapy drugs. Platinum drugs (cisplatin and carboplatin) can affect the auditory nerve and cause loss of hearing and tinnitus (ringing in the ears.) This damage is often permanent. The good news is they are also working on a drug which might help restore hearing. More power to them!

Tomorrow I would have to confess to the doctor what I did; I took unauthorized antibiotics. Do oncologists lop heads off unruly patients?

Thursday, December 29, 2011

Tis funny, but nothing changed.

Tuesday, I took Martha to work and then went and had my blood test. When I got home, I called the hospital. A nurse called back; she didn't know me from Eve, so she couldn't tell that my voice is not usually high soprano. I told her about my sinuses and ears (banging and ringing) and voice (I could sing high C, but then I probably would never be able to talk again) and she checked the results of my blood test on the computer. My immunity was borderline good; not bad. She would check with the doctor about antibiotics. And yes, Imodium for the runs and Preparation H (cream, not suppositories) for rectal bleeding were okay.

I did what I had been doing every day. I sat at the computer, playing games, drinking endless glasses of nasty tasting water and/or fruit juice, and once in a while snacking on meat and cheese, with applesauce, bananas, and ice cream for side dishes. Nothing else appealed. Swish with magic mouthwash every four hours and visit the toilet regularly. How often was regularly? Well, I used up a package of Cottonelle wipes, so I guess it comes out to about 10-15 times a day. But I was not dehydrated; my urine was not dark.

The nurse called back. The doctor agreed to give me an antibiotic. Thank God. I poured myself into the car and got my stuff from the pharmacy. Then I went back to my routine.

My ears and sinuses improved, but my voice did not. My throat was no longer bright red, but I had certifiable laryngitis. If I talked too much, my voice faded from soprano to squeak. I was sleeping better, but still not getting as much sleep as is optimum, so I tried to nap in the afternoon. My skin was dry, dry, dry. My lips were dry and I coated them with chapstick.

I finally stopped bleeding rectally (not going to swear it was hemorrhoids, but it probably was) yesterday. My anus stopped hurting so much thanks to the wipes, but now every delicate part covered by hair down there was uncomfortable, as if I had a yeast infection smeared all over. And no, I had no other signs of a yeast infection there, at least so far.

My taste buds improved, but were not normal. No, not normal. Vernors (a Detroit thing) tasted like regular ginger ale. It lost the something different that made it different from ginger ale. Broccoli was sweet as if I sprinkled sugar on it. Even chocolate tasted a little off. Water almost tasted like water—if you get your water from a dirty well. My tongue was sensitive, but no longer coated white. Instead it was an unhappy pink. I still swished magic mouthwash because without it, the thrush popped up again.

My gut—gastrointestinal tract—was okay, but felt uneasy. I still burped, but had not been nauseated. I could eat what I liked, but gravitated toward meat, potato, and vegetable dinners. Plain and simple. Did I realize I had eaten half a jar of peanut butter? It was slathered on low salt Ritz crackers, every bit. I was almost out of grape juice.

So, not much had changed. Except...

I woke up not feeling well. I didn't think I drank enough yesterday. So I slugged down grape juice water as fast as I could force it down. It made me feel better, but my taste buds slipped back into bad habits. There was a distinct chemical/metal taste in my mouth. I had been stubbornly eating one slice of pizza a day, although it was too spicy. Today, after drinking juice water like a drunken sailor, the second to last piece actually tasted good. Go figure.

Imodium, which usually makes me constipated after one dose, did not cut the runs. It was now all-out war waged with chewable pills. And I had not weighed myself. Breast cancer chemo tends to make one gain weight. My guess is it's because you feel better with something in your stomach.

A person in chemotherapy can have problems with their balance. This can be due to drugs affecting the brain or inner ear, dehydration, or plain old weakness. Losing balance can lead to less mobility, which can lead to more problems. The recommendation is to walk or do other light exercise (carefully,) breathe deeply to keep oxygen flowing, and keep rested, as in sleeping as well as possible.

My next chemo treatment was January 9th. Would I get a day or two of normal before then?

Saturday, December 31, 2011

New Year's Eve, everyone. Here's to a great new year.

So little to report. I no longer had diarrhea, but didn't have solid stools. I bet this was the new chemo norm. So, unless it got really bad, forget Imodium. I hated the thought of pouring more drugs into my system.

I had one of those lightening streaks of common sense: it must be thrush gone into my throat that ruined my voice. So I drank my magic mouthwash instead of spitting it out. Immediate improvement in the voice. Another call to the doctor's office confirmed this brilliant thought. "It'll just take longer to get rid of the thrush," the nurse said.

My ears were still bad. I dreaded the thought of my ears ringing for months, but the antibiotic didn't do much against it. The ringing must really be from the chemo. My sinus felt better, but I was getting frequent very tiny nosebleeds.

And now I had fissures (little cracks) in my tongue. Guess what caused them? Pick...

1) chemotherapy
2) thrush
3) the stress to my body

According to the Internet, all three apply. The cracks were superficial; they didn't go all the way through. They just made my tongue more sensitive and perhaps affected my taste buds. They looked ugly. I avoided sticking my tongue out at Rick.

But yesterday I woke up with what felt like my normal appetite. So, I figured that it took me a week and a half to recover from a chemo treatment. I sat like a bump on the log while the ball came down in Central Park and then headed for bed.

Can't say that I put any thought into my tumors being triple negative. At this point, it didn't matter. Cancer was cancer, treatment was treatment. Life and death squished to essentials.

Sunday, January 1, 2012

For the last several days, I had been getting vague aches and pains in the evening, mainly in my legs and arms in the vicinity of the elbow. Kind of like I was starting the achy flu. Ibuprofen pretty much took care of that.

The first time it happened, I stole Martha's ibuprofen. I am a Tylenol user, but the doctor had warned me to use ibuprofen if needed. It works against inflammation, a big thing with chemo. The first couple of times I took it, Rick asked what was wrong. After that, I noticed him noticing me taking it, but he didn't comment. Good man. I didn't want to hash out every twinge.

When I went to bed, I wanted to turn something to hash. The base of my spine throbbed. I had felt this once or twice at times associated with a difficult bowel movement, but those times, it lasted only a few seconds. This went on and on. I took ibuprofen and it didn't cut the discomfort, not one little bit. I lay in bed, my spine bump, bump, bumping, totally unable to get comfortable. Unable to sleep. You know the kind of discomfort that keeps you awake. Not quite full blooded pain, but miserable.

I think I fell asleep from exhaustion. This morning, my spine was still unhappy, but it slowly dissipated over the day. (Look for an explanation later. It was the side effect called bone and muscle ache.)

I no longer imagined hurdles to jump over in a mythical race. It was too depressing a scenario. Those hurdles kept getting closer together and higher. It was a struggle to jump them and I didn't want to discourage myself.

Tuesday, January 3, 2012

Took Martha to work and then stopped by Cottage Hospital for the blood work. They remembered me. By the time this testing every week was over, we'd be on going-out-to lunch terms.

Well, there goes the hair. No, it wasn't falling out all at once, but my pubic hair was globbing up the toilet paper. I didn't comb the hair on my head. I was trying to decide if I should just have Rick or Martha gently pull and get it over with rather than shedding all over the place. Or do it myself. It is these big decisions that hurt, you know. Looked forward to not having to shave; who needs razors, sucker? Not me!

I was keeping my eye on the goal: health.

A couple of my fingernails darkened. They can turn black, get loose, get thin, even fall off. Gross, but nails are an indicator of health or lack thereof. Another grin and bear it.

Except for thrush, which still plagued my throat, altered taste buds (not as bad as before, but not normal) and hair loss (incoming Yul Brenner) I felt pretty normal. A week from yesterday was the next chemo.

I could ignore the chest port. Believe it or not, Ripley, you do get used to it.

Thursday, January 5, 2012

I was to be at the hospital oncology department at 9 am Monday and in the Chemo room at 11. As if I had forgotten. (I had been switched from Tuesday to Monday.)

I no longer needed to shave under my arms. The hair on my head was intact, probably because I had not combed it. Deep psychological voodoo here. I ordered three turbans from the American Cancer Society's tlc catalog. Because I procrastinated, I used next day delivery; otherwise I would probably not have them until Monday. Needed one Saturday.

I had Martha finger comb my head; she said you couldn't really see a difference, but she's a big liar. My hair was much thinner and she kept brushing strands off her fingers into the wastebasket. A huge mound ended up in the wastebasket.

Almost all that came off was gray. If I kept my dark hair and lost the gray, I'd look incredibly weird. Can you see me walking down the street with a full head of hair in the back and nothing up front?

Short explanation—I turned gray at the temples, sides and top of my head, not so much in the back. Always laughed because it was what I could see that went first. Now, it was the gray going first. Still laughing with tears dripping from my heart.

Chemo can raise havoc with your skin. Dry skin is common; a good moisturizer does wonders; at least it might if you use it regularly. Hyper-pigmentation (darkening) may happen all over or in patches. Most of those changes fade away within months of finishing chemo. Photosensitivity, or increased reaction to sunlight, is another risk. Stay away from the sun—use a good, strong sunblock—wear protective clothing—avoid sunburn. Hives (itchy allergic bumps,) acne (good old zits,) Psoriasis (red patches with dry silvery scales,) or Purpura (purplish spots or blotches,) may plague you. How do you like that: seven plagues, just like Egypt.

Steven Johnson Syndrome may be the worst skin side effect. With it, you get extensive skin reactions up to blisters and erosions with flu-like symptoms. If you think this malady may have attacked you, call the doctor. It is too nasty to ignore and there is help available.

Any time you have pain, itching, blisters, or a temperature over 100°, call the doctor.

Actually, it doesn't hurt to call the doctor if you are worried about something or anything. Cancer treatment is so complicated, anything that bothers you may be rooted in something the doctor needs to know about and can treat.

Chemotherapy Cycle 2

Tuesday, January 10, 2012

Yesterday began Cycle 2 of my chemotherapy. In other words, I had to go in for the second time for them to dump poison into my system. I had to be at Henry Ford Hospital at 9 to see the doctor, so Rick took Martha to work and then came back for me. It let me sleep a little longer.

It didn't take long to get ready—clean up, dress, and grab the bag I prepared the night before. It held my binder of information and my new Kindle. Bravely, I did not wear a hat, although I crammed one in the bag.

When I checked in, they weighed me, checked my blood pressure and temperature, and did a blood test. The girl drew my blood using the chest port, which was balky. It would stop and start, stop and start. She kept flushing it with saline and finally it behaved. Surprise, surprise, she didn't take the IV out, but left it hanging, ready for the chemo session at 11, covered with that huge clear band-aid (which did not hurt when it was removed.) It was bothersome when I walked, but didn't actively hurt.

I lost ten pounds in three weeks. No one minded.

First I saw a junior doctor, who took the list of side effects I had suffered. Rick said later that I seemed to fluster him—the guy probably wasn't used to efficient women. My whole point was to make sure I didn't miss anything important.

Yes, I could take Naproxen for my back; just try not to take a lot of it. Thank God for small favors! Adding the headaches I get from my persnickety back to the junk I dealt with via chemo would make me want to die. Figuratively, not literally.

My blood numbers were respectable. Immunity, which was critical, was elevated, he thought from the Dexamethasone I took on Sunday. It's a steroid, bad for my eyes, but great for everything else. Maybe it would turn me into Superwoman.

After a long wait, I saw the big doctor. Not Dr. Medica; she was off doing intensive work at two hospitals. When they are scheduled for that, they don't do the Breast Cancer Clinic. Hey, something has to go. So, I saw this other guy. The important thing was he cleared me for the chemo treatment.

So Rick and I were free for 45 minutes. We went outside and had a cigarette, then stopped at the coffee shop. I got apple juice, a banana and a cranberry muffin; he got his coffee. Then we took the elevator to Floor 13 and the clinic. I scarfed the banana down in the waiting room and turned on my Kindle.

I was a pro in the Chemo room. I knew where everything was and I knew the basic procedures. I had a different nurse—she had four kids, most in some kind of sports, and she was jealous of my Kindle. She had seen HBO's True Blood series, and that was what I was watching. I hoped that watching a show distracted me better than reading did before. The sounds of the chemotherapy room vaguely disturbed me. Not disturbed as in momentarily distracted me, but disturbed as in bothered me.

Taking a trick from the Internet, I poured apple juice over ice and made sure to keep ice rolling around my mouth the first few minutes of each drug entering my body through the IV. Didn't know if it would help with my mouth, but the thought is the cold constricts the cells in the mouth, keeping the drugs from going there as much. The nurse knew of the idea, but she had never heard it was proven. It didn't hurt to try. Sure would like it if water didn't taste like dirt, not to mention every kind of food.

I used the hospital pharmacy to get more magic mouthwash. The nurse or doctor called down the prescription and they delivered it to me in the Chemo room. This time I got modified magic mouthwash. There was no information as to what was in it; I assumed it was a stronger thrush killer. I wouldn't bother to ask unless I had problems with it.

I also asked for the cream (which turned out to be Lidocaine and Prilocaine) that deadens the area around the chest port. I didn't mind the poke of the IV going in; it was walking around with it hanging from me that was a bit uncomfortable. The nurse advised me to slather the Lidocaine on really thick an hour before my appointment, and put a bit of plastic wrap over it so it soaked into my skin, not into my shirt. (I pinned a baggie to the inside of my shirt.) Only used it once; the benefits of the deadening did not outweigh the bother of smearing.

Rick made a food run. We both got ham and Swiss cheese sandwiches on wheat. My appetite was amazing. He read his book and I got through two and a half episodes of True Blood before I was done with chemo at 2 pm.

Like the first treatment, it was the Cytoxan that I could taste in my mouth. Also, partway through that dose, I suddenly got really tired, ready for a nap. I pushed through it and we went home.

I nibbled my way through the afternoon. For dinner, we had spaghetti—not my choice because of the acidity of the tomato sauce, but Rick was cooking and he likes spaghetti. I didn't eat a lot of it, but I did have chocolate ice cream for dessert. Went to bed at 11:30 after dozing in the chair for an hour.

This morning, I felt fine, with one BIG exception. My right hand (except the index finger and thumb) was a bit tingly and numb. My own diagnosis was neuropathy. Didn't want it, especially on the side that does all the work. I called the doctor's office and talked to a nurse. She didn't have any suggestions: if it got too painful to live with, go to the Emergency Room. Otherwise, make sure I tell the doctor about it before my next chemo. She might want to adjust the dose.

Hi, Internet. It is properly called peripheral neuropathy. What happens is the chemo drugs don't just attack the cancer; they also go after other things in the body. Some of those things are nerve endings, especially the nerves for the fingers and toes. They are so small, it makes sense they would get messed up. Usually it will be in both fingers or both toes, not just on one side. If it's in the fingers or toes, it can gradually move upward as if you are donning imaginary stockings or gloves. It can also attack the bowels, causing constipation or intestinal blockage, or bother the face (causing drooling, et cetera,) back, or chest.

It can feel like numbness, tingling, burning, the loss of sensation of touch, weakness, or difficulty using the part affected. I knew from others that if it is in your fingers, it can make it difficult or impossible to button buttons, zip zippers, tie shoelaces—it can make you totally miserable and even disabled.

The people most at risk of getting neuropathy during chemo treatment are diabetics, alcoholics, those who are severely malnourished, and those poor suckers who have been there and done that before. Overall, 30-40% of people who get hooked to a chemotherapy IV get neuropathy. It is one of the common reasons for giving up chemo.

According to the sites I visited, neuropathy may appear suddenly. The sensation usually builds gradually and can get worse with each chemo treatment. It is usually strongest right after chemo, but lessens before the next treatment. It is unpredictable; it comes and goes without warning.

It can disappear, only to return years later. Sometimes it stays the same strength, other times it can be worse or lighter in symptoms.

So what can you do about it? First, tell the doctor, follow his or her instructions, and be active in decisions regarding treatment versus quality of life. Sometimes, the symptoms can be lessened by lowering the dose of chemotherapy or temporarily stopping it, which can lessen the pain within a few weeks. There are drugs to take, but they have their own side effects, so taking them you might be between the devil and the deep blue sea. And they don't always work. For some people, the symptoms last for months, years, or forever.

Make sure you rest. Rest the affected part, get plenty of sleep, if you can. Neuropathy can hurt so much you have trouble sleeping. Protect the poor body part: avoid extremes of temperature, be careful that you don't injure it. Watch out for infection. If it is fingers or toes, wear good thick socks and soft-soled shoes or wear gloves when washing dishes or gardening. Gardening? I can't imagine gardening while going through chemo.

Get a supply of vitamins in the B-complex family. The B vitamins support your nerves.

For comfort: massage, lotions and creams, even splints to support the poor baby. Deep breathing, relaxation and guided imagery might help with the pain.

If you get constipated, eat high fiber foods and drink two to three quarts of non-alcoholic fluids a day. Exercise twenty to thirty minutes—walking is convenient—anything and everything to keep your bowels moving. If the doctor gives you a regimen to follow, make sure you follow it exactly. After all, intestinal blockage can kill you.

Your doctor might send you to physical therapy, put you in a brace or splint, and if the neuropathy gets bad enough, you might need biofeedback, acupuncture, or transcutaneous nerve stimulation (TENS)—stimulation of the nerves with electric current. Don't do it yourself! Sticking your afflicted finger into the electric socket won't do the job.

By midafternoon, my hand felt pretty normal. Martha stopped at the drug store after work and talked to the pharmacist about B-Complex vitamins. He advised against buying them since I was already taking Centrum Silver, which has the B's in it. But... Centrum doesn't have a high dose of B vitamins and more Internet surfing said maybe I wanted to get them anyway.

Thursday, January 12, 2012

Woke up feeling yucky, like I was getting the flu. The magic mouthwash had my mouth under control; food and water didn't taste great, but it wasn't like eating dirt. (So maybe sucking ice when the IV drip starts does help.) Breakfast was three sticks of string cheese, grape juice and chocolate donuts for taste. I popped some Advil (it is an ibuprofen,) ate, and vegged out.

Plenty of people push through and lead an active life while doing chemotherapy, but I didn't have to. I could be a miserable vegetable if I wanted.

My ears were blocking up. I put in a call in to Dr. Sanatio. Hopefully he would agree to give me an antibiotic.

Martha ran her hands through my hair and removed more. Lots more. You would not believe how falling out hair can fill a trash can unless you see it for yourself. Turbans and hats were no longer a fashion statement. I needed them.

Sunday, January 15, 2012

Do you think that you are going to need help getting through chemotherapy? Cooking, cleaning, or laundry (or all of the above) may be too much for you. You might be shaky. You might even be bedridden. If you live alone, magnify difficulties because having a spouse, significant other, or child around on a daily basis might ease your burden. They can take up the slack.

Ok. You need help. Do you have any idea how much help is available out there? Where do you find it?

First, neighbors, friends, and relatives might be eager, willing, and able to help. They can run to the store for you; they might do anything and everything that needs doing. But they don't know you need help until you cry SOS.

If they require payment, work something out. Handing over your first born child is a dandy way to pay debts, but chances are they only need a couple of bucks to put gas in the car or a blank check made out to the grocery store. If you feel obligated, promise yourself to search out the perfect birthday or Christmas present once you are back on your feet.

Try to spread requests for assistance around; any one person is just too darn busy to become your slave for several months.

Low on available neighbors and relatives?

The Livestrong Foundation suggests:
- Contact a local cancer organization or hospital.
- Search online for a keyword and your area. Example: food banks, Austin, Texas.
- Read the government and business sections of the phone book. (This can be overwhelming. Try looking for senior citizen agencies.)
- Call a social worker or the Department of Health and Human Services in your area.
- Call the United Way helpline. Dial 211.
- How about the National Cancer Institute?
- Meals On Wheels can cook.
- Visiting Angels can help you get dressed, do light housekeeping, etc. Ask, and ye shall receive.

Thursday, January 19, 2012

Now I knew pretty well how my body dealt with chemotherapy. It could be worse. Here are the ways I counted the days:

I didn't get nauseated. That was a blessing.

I did get thrush. It popped up right away and didn't go away without concerted attack by medicine. My voice was still not right; my vocal cords must have been irritated. The thrush fell out of my mouth in a rush after about seven days of modified magic mouthwash. My tongue was left red, sensitive, sore in spots, but that eased up. It did mess up my taste buds. Perhaps someday food would taste as it should. My lips got a coating of a good strong chapstick at bedtime; I could use it during the day, but disliked the feel. I needed that chapstick.

I tended toward diarrhea. It was controllable, but using toilet paper instead of wipes, my rear got sore right away. I took one Imodium and promptly got constipated, followed by more diarrhea, so I gave up treating it. Bouncing between loose as a goose and tighty mighty wasn't worth the discomfort. Wipes kept hemorrhoids under control. I pretty much dropped toilet paper from my list of friends. My new buddy was Cottonelle wipes.

This is important, folks! Infection is a problem when your immune system is depressed. The open sores that are hemorrhoids can get infected very easily. Just think how that would feel.

Hair was still falling off my head. I looked like a direct descendant of Scrooge and Betelgeuse. Straggly, flyaway, sticking out and laying every which way hair, and my scalp was sensitive. It got itchy. I didn't like to look at my head. And no, I was never so handsome as Yul Brynner or Captain Jean Luc Picard of the Enterprise. My head is shaped like a pear.

Turbans from the tlc catalog did not look on me as they looked on the models. The twists they sell would be fine if the design went all the way around, but my head is LARGE and I had a good four inches of cloth covered Velcro at the back of my head, rather than a pretty twist. I didn't look at it, but I knew that stretch of Velcro defeated pretty. My daughter bought several cloth headbands the same idea as the Cancer Society's twist, but softer and more forgiving in the back. They made the turbans wearable.

I could do scarves, but never used them before and getting them tied and looking pretty was more work than I had energy to put in. I never considered a wig, though that was an option.

The end result was that I only wore a hat at home when my ears got cold; most of the day (and night) I put up with a cool head. Pity my husband and daughter having to gaze at my egghead. It's a good thing they love me for more than my looks. Going out, I wore whatever I must. I had visions of little kids running screaming if I didn't have something on my head.

My temperature was in the mid 97's. When it was in the mid 98's, I felt like I had a fever. The closest I came to normal—98.6—was 98.5 and I was sweating as if I had run a mile. Just took my temp and it was 97.4°. Yes, my temperature tends to go down when I don't feel well. It is one of the ways I know if I have a low grade infection. So I treated myself as if I was an invalid.

My appetite was down for several days after the second chemo treatment, but then it went to fairly normal. Because I learned to manage my mouth better and figured out what pleased my sickly taste buds, I was eating more normally, but I leaned toward very simple meals. My husband put pepper in scrambled eggs and I could taste it and wanted to sneeze. No, he didn't pour a teaspoon in, but I requested he skip seasonings.

I was losing weight, but more slowly. After the first chemo, I lost perhaps half a pound a day; now it was probably a few ounces. If I stopped eating ice cream I might lose more, but I was addicted to a mouth soothing doesn't taste like dirt menu.

It finally dawned on me that my sinuses were extremely dry. Maybe that was why I was getting bloody nose after bloody nose, though there wasn't much blood. I sprayed Ocean up my nostrils several times a day, which soothed the savage beast. In case you didn't know, Ocean is an over-the-counter liquid that you use when your nose gets too dry, like when you are on an airplane with all that recycled dry air assaulting you. It is formulated to be like the natural moisture in your sinuses.

The last couple of days, my nose was runny. Runny is a huge plus versus stuffy, though my bad sinus got stuffy. No surprise that a runny nose is a side effect of the drugs, even when you have a sinus infection. Dr. Sanatio was kind enough to issue a prescription for antibiotic. I wanted to get his opinion on why it was now my ears bothering me more than the sinus. It wasn't tinnitus; it was clogged ears.

How many people have chronic conditions to deal with while they fight cancer? If you know how to pacify your chronic problem, then you are a step ahead—just be ready to up the ante and find alternative therapies and shifts in attack. Drugs you commonly take might fight with the chemo drugs, and those take precedence. Creativity may be required. You may have to substitute something that works less well for something that works great.

I had several achy days after the second chemo. My thighs and knees were the main culprits, although my arms just above the elbows twinged. I kept up with ibuprofen and made it through, although once or twice I considered Tylenol 3. The base of my spine didn't throb this time.

This is bone and muscle ache and isn't to be ignored, as neglecting to treat it can encourage it to get worse. Arthralgias is the medical term. Although people call it bone pain, it is probably due to chemoed nerves. (If you have metastasized cancer, it might be the bone itself.) It can show up as redness or swelling around a joint like an elbow or ankle. It might cause you to run a fever or have chills. And of course, you will have pain—either constant or coming and going, sharp or dull. The advice is to fight back before it becomes overwhelming.

Checking the Internet, some people had it at the base of the spine, as I did during Cycle 1. Others reported it starting there and traveling up the spine, ending in a pounding headache, so I had it easy. It can hit the jaw or the hips. It can hit anywhere. It can be just a dull achy feeling or pain so bad that Vicodin doesn't stop it. Hopefully it is a transitory thing, going away, as my aches did. For some, though, the pain continues after chemo ends.

Many people breathe lightly when pain hits them. Don't do this; it is nonproductive. Keep breathing deeply. Good strong breathing circulates oxygen and staves off infection. Exercise without killing yourself. A warm compress (washcloth dipped in warm water and wrung out) might relieve symptoms. Ibuprofen may calm it down. Physical therapy might be called for.

As with all symptoms and side effects, mention it to your doctor and see what he says. There might be a medication that will ease the pain. A support group might help you live with it. What won't help is whining and moaning. That will just focus your attention on the misery. Out of mind is out of sight.

On a related topic, be aware that chemotherapy can cause arthritis to begin or worsen, but the experts assure us it is usually self-limiting. It goes away. Then again, they use chemotherapy to treat arthritis.

One person in a chat room got the dilemma out clearly: "... every blasted drug you take puts a burden on the organs that are most responsible for clearing toxins out of your body—liver and kidney. Those are the same organs that produce the chemicals that manage to keep your system balanced... and keep anger, depression, pain, etc., under control. They have a hard time, and everything has a hard time." Inflammation is the culprit for many of the aches and pains chemo patients suffer. Get the inflammation down and the discomfort should ease.

I was sleeping better. So there.

My fingernails were darkening at the cuticle. Both thumbs looked as if I used a magic marker on them and only half-washed the ink off. I decided to pretend to be Goth. The dark nails were developing a ditch going across them—a depression. It was most pronounced on the thumbs, which were also the darkest. And my fingernails were sensitive. I needed to cut them short in order to type. Interesting that my toenails were fine.

Nails can become brittle and crack or break, going so far as to fall off during chemo. I was told that Henry Ford Health System's Dermatology Department is pretty good at giving manicures on mangled nails. My daughter offered to put nail polish on, but I hesitated. Yes, my hands would look better, but then the polish would chip, I would have to use nail polish remover, and what would those chemicals do on top of everything else? The trusty Internet says to avoid using polish unless you have the type of nails that get stronger under its influence. Sounds like it is personal preference here, ladies. Paint away, but if your nails are affected greatly, check with your oncologist about care.

If you are addicted to manicures, go easy and have the manicurist sterilize the instruments. They are a prime candidate for introducing bacteria into the body, and your chemoed immune system can't handle it. God forbid you use fake nails and pull your real nails off when you remove them.

I scratched an itch on the underside of my forearm. Lo and behold, I had to hold a Kleenex over the spot for a couple of minutes until it stopped bleeding. I was not sure if I had a pimple there or what. Be aware of problems with bleeding and mention it to your oncologist. It is probably because your blood counts are screwed up from the chemo.

Use common sense. You don't want to seriously cut yourself instead of a carrot and bleed to death. (Not a joke. Bleeding can be a problem.) Likewise, I absently scratched a pimple on my face (which popped up out of nowhere) and it bled like a stuck pig. I tried to be more conscious of unconscious and random scratching. My skin was drier, thus itchier. Invest in a good moisturizer. The skin can get so dry it cracks—and the cracks get infected.

My forehead peeled with both chemo treatments. Don't ask me to explain it. Didn't understand, just flaked peeling skin off and shrugged.

Without consulting the doctor, I started taking Super B-Complex vitamins along with my Centrum Silvers. The B vitamins support nerves, as in tingling and numb finger and toe nerves. It might be a waste of money, swallowing the extra B vitamins, because the body doesn't absorb them from pills efficiently, but I was determined to try to help my nerves. I did not want my hands crippled by neuropathy. I would not exceed the dosage on the vitamins—too much B can be as bad or worse than not enough. And I would discuss it with the oncologist.

Don't forget the weekly blood test. It only took a few minutes since I managed to be at the lab when there was no one else there.

I could tell when I needed to drink more water. I would taste the chemicals in my mouth more. Nasty. Soda pop still tasted strange. I preferred purple grape juice and added apple juice for variety. Apple was a bit acidic at times; I could feel the acid on my lips. Orange was downright unpleasant. Martha had the brilliant idea to buy bottled water. Ahh, it did taste better than tap water. Not great, but better.

Dehydration is an enemy. I did well drinking the first week, but slacked off the second. I am a sipper, not a gulper, but needed to gulp. Thanks for the reminder. My glass was empty.

The medical bills were amusing. A lab pathology bill from November (from the lumpectomy) was $1,800. I didn't have to pay a cent and Blue Cross paid $342. It is a wonder the medical community doesn't go bankrupt. You know some guy spent a good bit of time peering at my tumor through a microscope. How much of the $342 did he get? How much paid for the microscope, heat, lights, and telephone? Add nurses, clerks, vacuuming the rug in the reception room, hiring snow plows for the parking lot. No, they were not getting rich off me.

Then again, I had an echocardiogram. It was one technician, a few minutes hooked up to a machine. The charge was $1,300, of which insurance paid $444 and I had to pay $170. A PET scan cost twice as much as a MRI.

$6,000? Wow. It looked like a mammogram was an affordable $300.

I arranged to pay Henry Ford Health System $100 per month for keeping me alive and Macomb Hospital $50 per month for carving a smiley face in my boob. My food budget was wacko from feeding husband and daughter while satisfying my special needs.

Monday, January 23, 2012

It is getting tougher, and more dangerous, Mr. Cancer. The funny thing is you don't seem so real to me anymore. I feel like I am shadow boxing—fighting nothing. In the back of my mind is the knowledge that what I am doing is very important, life sustaining, but it doesn't have such an impact on my emotions. Guess I am too busy doing what I have to do.

Makes sense—a person can't spend months on the knife edge. At some point, one has to slide down off the edge and hope one makes it to solid ground without too much damage. Danger, a threat to one's life, becomes secondary to living, even if the living isn't high quality at the moment.

That was more than enough philosophizing. I had a report to make.

This week was not fun. Today, I woke up at 5 am with boggy sinuses and unhappy ears. This is while I was taking antibiotics, mind. Obviously, my immune system was not at its peak.

Of course, I couldn't get back to sleep. I read until Rick and Martha roused. The plan was for me to take Martha to work and then go get my weekly blood test, return a healed computer to a client, and run errands. Hopefully I could make an appointment to talk to Dr. Sanatio. He might have ideas for subordinating an aching head. Don't ask why I set such an ambitious schedule for the day. I must have been nuts.

It wasn't until I was ready to go out the door that I looked out the window. What to my wondering eyes did appear, but my miniature silver Sunfire sleigh with three perfectly good tires and one extremely flat tire. Damn. Martha called in to tell whomever that she would be late to work and I called a tow truck.

I did my duty and made an appointment to see Dr. Sanatio in the afternoon. Then we sat around for an hour until the tow truck arrived. The guy pulled the flat off the car, put some air in it, and checked for something obvious like a nail embedded in it. Nothing. So he put the spare tire on, threw the flat in my trunk, got paid, and we left.

Already I felt low on energy. Driving carefully so I didn't do in the spare tire, I watched for potholes, of which the Detroit area had more than its share, and slowed down for railroad tracks (two sets in my way.) But Martha got to work, I got the computer back to the client, up and running like a dream, and realized I had to eat. Like right now. And I had one hour until I had to be at the doctor's office. That meant McDonald's. Not the healthiest meal, but a quarter pounder with cheese and some fries filled my stomach. Too bad Coke tasted like pure carbonation; I had to pretend it had flavor. Chalk up another drink ruined by chemo mouth.

Dr. Sanatio didn't have any ideas to make me feel better. Bless him, he did agree to dispense antibiotics as needed. I would try not to abuse the privilege, but I had to drag my head through chemo somehow. Couldn't make it through anything if my sinus was infected and my ears hurt. After I got done with treatment, I would go back to dealing with lawless sinuses in a more sensible and holistic manner.

Priorities. Save my life and then worry about irritations. Dr. Sanatio did think that I was dealing well with chemo and eased my mind about my temperature. It's okay to hover around 97°. Don't worry unless I went below 96°.

Leaving the doctor's office at 2 pm, my eyes felt like boiled onions with dirt thrown in. Better get the blood test done before I fell over. I didn't have any stamina. I headed for Cottage Hospital—the radio told me not to take the expressway. I saved some time avoiding the accident that snarled the road.

Blood test done, my car demanded I take the flat tire to Grosse Pointe Shell. They have long been our choice for car repairs. They don't cheat, they don't treat me like a stupid woman. Doug, the owner, has the patience of Job with our poor car. Tired I might be, but I couldn't ignore the flat. I left it at Grosse Pointe Shell. They would fix it and I would come back to have it put back on.

Finally, I could go home. I was too tired to run errands. I sat and watched TV, not something I usually do during the day, at least when I am healthy.

I had to pick Martha up from work so I resisted taking a nap. She kindly ordered carry-out so no one had to cook. Bottle washing was handled by the dishwasher. I checked with Grosse Pointe Shell; they had not found anything wrong with the tire. Left it there overnight to be sure.

The newest side effect was eye tics; they were worse when I was tired. With the full day I had just put in, I felt like a Regency era debutante fluttering her eyelashes at the handsome bachelor Duke. Or the whore winking at him.

Cancer Genetics

Tuesday, January 24, 2012

My appointment with the Cancer Genetics Program was at 8 am. The Sunfire limped on the skinny little spare tire to Greektown, taking Martha to work, and then up to New Center One on East Grand Boulevard, down the street from the hospital. Once there, seated across the table from a geneticist, I realized I was apprehensive.

Let's go over the reasons for my being there:
1) With my strong family history of breast cancer (Mom, aunt, Grandma and Grandma's cousin—and as I found out later, Grandma's mother) there was a chance I carried the breast cancer genes, technically known as BRCA1 and BRCA2. For the sake of my daughters, not to mention other family members, I wanted to know if I had them. If I did, they might also. Forewarned is ammunition.
2) My oncologist wanted to know if I carried the breast cancer genes. If I did, she might change my treatment plan.

Why was I apprehensive? Refer to 1 and 2 above.

The geneticist, a very nice woman named Dr. C—(you don't think I remembered her name, do you?) took my family history. She'd had lots of practice drawing genealogy charts; once we got done with four generations, it was still neat and readable.

The four generations were my
- daughters, sons (none,) nieces and nephews
- brothers, sisters (none,) and cousins
- parents, aunts and uncles
- and grandparents

She asked about learning and physical disabilities, general health, causes of death, and ages of death. Lalie, my grandmother's cousin who had breast cancer in the 1920's, didn't matter for the chart. Dr. C—wrote her off to the side. She might not matter, but Dr. C—still found her significant. Maybe she was humoring me and didn't care about Lalie, but I did.

After she got the family information, Dr. C—started explaining BRCA genes. They are mutations (changes) on two genes, one on Chromosome 13 and the other on Chromosome 17. Everyone has the two genes, but not everyone has the mutations. The experts think that these two mangled genes account for 7% of all breast cancers and 10% of ovarian cancers. Not very big percentages, but the numbers represent around 16,000 people a year.

The BRCA genes are more complicated than that, but I am not the person to go to for information. The experts understand BRCA better than I ever could.

My advice would be that if breast cancer seems to run in your family, find out if you can be tested. At the Henry Ford Health System Cancer Genetics program, you have to already have cancer to be tested, but if you test positive for BRCA, your family members become eligible to be tested. And don't just think females. Men can get breast cancer also. Add ovarian, pancreatic, and prostate cancers to the list that BRCA is thought to influence, and you find lots of reasons to be tested.

How do BRCA genes get passed on? To make a complicated science simple, all men and women have two sets of each chromosome. They pass on half of those sets to their baby. Look at the chart below. The X's, Z's and H's, etc. represent chromosomes.

	Father	Mother	Baby
Chromosome 13	X O	Z Y	X Y
Chromosome 17	T W	C H	W C

As you can see, Baby got her genes as a random mix from Mom and Dad. Both parents might have escaped having BRCA mutilated genes or one or both of them have bad BRCA genes. Say that Dad's X has BRCA1; he passed it on to Baby. But if Dad's X is clean and O has BRCA1, Baby is in the clear. Ditto with Mom's chromosomes and the same scenario holds for BRCA2. Either Baby got BRCA or she didn't.

It counts for boys as well as girls; boys can inherit mangled BRCA genes and develop cancer. If Dad or Mom has a mutation, there is a 50% chance of Baby getting it. The only way Baby is absolutely doomed to get BRCA is if one of the parent's chromosomes has double mutations (for example Dad's X and O both have BRCA.) Then Baby is sure to get a bad gene.

This counts for all their children, if they have one or if they have ten. Some or all of their kids might inherit BRCA.

A lot of family members getting breast cancer suggests they might carry the cockeyed BRCA genes. But with the way genetics works, you can't assume you have them. That is what testing is for.

Don't panic. Having a BRCA gene doesn't automatically say you will get cancer. It means that you have a higher risk of getting cancer. If your mom and grandma have diabetes, you know you should be careful about how you eat, etc., since you are more likely to develop diabetes, right? Same thing with breast cancer. There are things you can do to protect yourself, if only to make sure you catch the cancer early, when it is easier to cure.

And no, you don't have to go to the extreme of having healthy breasts amputated to avoid cancer. Some high profile women have done that, but I think it is cutting off your breast to spite your face. How could they let something control them this much? Remember, this is my uninformed opinion. No one discussed mastectomies with me and I didn't look this up on the Internet. Maybe those women had such strong histories that cancer was a foregone conclusion... No, I still don't understand it. Just know it can be done, okay?

There are two parts to the genetic test for BRCA, both done with a vial of blood supplied by the person being tested. I'd been giving my blood away recklessly, why not one more?

The first test, a full sequence analysis, costs over $4,000. Dr. C— assured me that the company doing the testing is not inflating the price. It is labor intensive, detailed work locating Chromosomes 13 and 17, finding the correct genes on the chromosomes, and figuring out if they are normal or mutated. The analogy is that with the first test, if genes are a book, the lab is spell checking the whole book. A misspelled word is mutated.

The second part of the test is a gene rearrangement test. If the genes are a book, this time the lab looks to see if the chapters of the book are out of order. If Chapter Three comes after Chapter Ten, the gene is mutated. That test costs $700-800.

The geneticists decide if one or both tests are done. Pray (check!) that your insurance covers the testing; not all do. I was lucky. HAP, my new insurance carrier, covered the full cost.

The results would either be negative (no BRCA genes,) positive (I had BRCA,) or inconclusive (I had genes that were not "normal," but the changes were different than the known BRCA mutations.) About 5% of the people tested get inconclusive results, called "variants of uncertain clinical significance." Further research might be able to figure out if these changes are bad cancer-wise, or benign (having nothing to do with cancer.)

I would have to go back to get the results; they wanted to sit down with me and go over them. I would also get a written report.

The Cancer Genetics Program wanted me to let them know if I moved, so if my BRCA report was changed by research down the road, they could contact me. If someone else in the family developed cancer, I should let them know. Although I was not expressly told so, I was sure my test results would be used in mutation research, which is a boon to the future.

In case you are tearing your hair out about mutations, don't think you are going to turn into a giant ant and eat New York City. Mutations are to be expected; they are a part of the human race evolving. Yes, some mutations are bad, but they can be good. Your baby could be born with a mutation that made it immune to the common cold. That would be one to cheer about.

Mutations are not incredibly rare. An example: genealogy researchers use DNA testing to figure out family relationships. Test men who have the same last name and think they might be related (using a special kit, they swab the inside of their mouth to get DNA and send it in.) The results can tell if you share a common ancestor. Test enough people with the same last name and you can start to sort out families.

I have Sarah Howman married to Joseph Keeler—they are my three times great-grandparents. One of Sarah's relatives shows a mutation. How did they find it? There were two brothers—a descendant of one brother was tested and has one DNA, but a descendant of the other brother who was tested has something different. No one knows what the mutation does—it is one number in a long string of numbers—but it is there.

By the way, the same DNA tests gave us Sarah Howman's ancestry. It fit this obscure family together so that, allowing for one questionable generation where the father could be one of two brothers (not the DNA mutated brothers,) you can trace Sarah's family back to 1620's Wurttemberg, Germany. Pretty neat, huh? All it took was a bunch of men with surnames in variations of Hammann undergoing DNA testing, including five men in my extended family, none of whom I know.

I'd better move away from genealogy. I could run on for a long time and bore you to death. Although I do suggest you learn your genealogy for at least four generations so you can tell the geneticist ages and causes of death for your parents, grandparents and maybe great-grandparents as well as your descendants. If you know the info, write it down so your kids and grandkids have it. The chances of them remembering that your grandmother died of breast cancer at age 72 drops as time goes on.

I donated a vial of blood to be sent to the lab and left. So, there you have the first visit to the Cancer Genetics Program.

Martha didn't feel well. She thought she was coming down with the flu. I avoided her and she avoided me. I did not need to be sick. With my compromised immune system, I could become really sick. I could miss my chemo treatment next Monday, which could make the whole chemo thing not work as well, which could make me get cancer again, which could... You get the idea.

Thanks for the memories

- In 400 BC, Hippocrates described breast cancer as a humoral disease caused by black bile or melancholia. He labeled it karkinos, meaning "crab," because tumors seemed to have tentacles that looked like crab legs. Imagine how big the tumor must have been for him to see legs.
- In 180 AD, a Greek, Leonides, is credited as the first doctor to surgically remove a breast.
- An Islamic surgeon from William the Conqueror's time (1066 and all that) wrote that he did not know anyone who had been able to cure breast cancer.
- A Dutchman performed lumpectomies in the 17th century.
- In 1810, the daughter of John and Abigail Adams, Abigail "Nabby" Adams Smith was diagnosed with breast cancer. She underwent a grueling mastectomy without anesthesia, but died a short time later.
- Fanny Burney, author of Camelia, was operated on for you know what by Napoleon's surgeons for almost four hours without any anesthesia beyond a wine cordial. She lived 29 years longer but never forgot that she screamed continuously for four hours.
- The first operation to use anesthesia was a breast cancer surgery.
- The first radiation treatments were at the turn of the 20th century.
- Research in 1975 led to the discovery of BRCA genes.

Friday, January 27, 2012

Hey, Cancer, you there? Listen up, I've got something to tell you.

You are laughing up your sleeve aren't you. "Stupid woman," you're saying, "You don't have a clue yet how nasty I can get."

Yeah, so maybe I didn't quite get the whole thing. Concepts are one thing, reality is something different. Chemotherapy poisons your body. I knew what that meant, but I didn't know. Well, now I do. Don't try that trick again, Cancer. I'm wise to you.

Today, my mouth bled when I brushed my teeth. Couldn't see where the blood was coming from if not from the gum line, but obviously I would have to be gentler. A soft toothbrush is sometimes not soft enough. The experts suggest softening the brush in warm water before using it or even switching to gauze pads. So be it.

I was starting a new (improved?) hemorrhoid. So I could bleed from both ends. How delightful. At least I knew it was a hemorrhoid. Any bleeding from that end of the body that can't be firmly identified as a hemorrhoid merits a call to the doctor. Heavy bleeding from that end means an immediate call. Ditto if you throw up blood. Things like the colon and the esophagus can be irritated by chemo and require emergency attention.

Last night, my ears woke me up. Especially the right ear, the one closest to the sinus that can't behave. That sinus was heavy, working up a good snit, and the ear was cheering it on. Well, I fixed that when I went to see Dr. Sanatio the other day. I had a prescription waiting at the pharmacy; Martha (who was looking and sounding better) went to pick it up.

So I had more antibiotic. If nothing else, the pills would keep my head down to a dull roar.

I didn't feel good. I just did not feel good in any way.

I might spend the next few months sicker than a homeless dog with mange, fleas, ticks, and the beginnings of lockjaw, but I would not quit chemo. Nope, I'd make every appointment without fail. I'd tell the doctors to admit me to the hospital and pour more antibiotics in my veins if necessary, but I wouldn't quit chemo.

But I felt as sick as a dog that had had an untreated sinus infection for months. I was just as snarly, too.

No matter what, I will survive you, Mr. Cancer. You are going to shrivel and die. Not me, you.

Chemotherapy Cycle 3

Tuesday, January 31, 2012

The town was abuzz over a local murder. I'd lived in Grosse Pointe all my life and could count the number of murders there on one hand. So, yes, the town was buzzing over Jane Bashara's murder. I felt sorry for her children and sorry for her husband provided he wasn't the murderer. We would see what the police came up with. Rick was interested; I was more interested in chemotherapy and its effects on the human body.

Yesterday was my third chemo treatment. Made for a long day and delays made this one longer. My appointment with the doctor was for 10:20 rather than 9:00; while it made getting to the hospital simpler, considering a family that doesn't like getting up with the sun, it turned out to be less desirable considering doctors' schedules.

Rick and I were there on time, but the doctor was running late. More than an hour late. Finally, the staff decided to have me see a different doctor. She turned out to be Dr. Medica, the oncologist in charge of my case.

As usual, I had a list of the symptoms I suffered through the second chemo cycle, as well as a few questions. Here is the list:

- The chest port felt funny over the weekend.
- Could I take Super B Vitamin Complex as well as regular vitamins?
- Getting antibiotics from Dr. Sanatio. Ok?
- Thrush: what is in the modified mouthwash? Could I swallow it?
- Eye tics almost continuous, as well as a few on the tip of my tongue (which felt weird.)
- Temperature going low.
- Sunday night, after taking Dexamethasone, I suffered frequent urination. Went at least five times before going to bed; a healthy amount of nearly clear urine each time.

Question 1 was answered by the nurse who hooked up the IV for the chemo and drew blood. The chest port had tipped toward my sternum. It probably happened because I slept funny Friday night, curled up with my right arm draped over my chest. She held it straighter and it worked fine. They wouldn't do anything about it unless it didn't work.

Dr. Medica was highly in favor of me taking the Super B Complex vitamins. If it was such a good idea, they should put the recommendation in their black notebook. She also approved of Dr. Sanatio handling my sinus and ear problems; she thought he was more versed in the situation, which was perfectly true. He had spent more than five years dealing with my sinus infections and whining. I should call the Breast Cancer clinic only if I had difficulties with him.

It wasn't thrush attacking my mouth so much as it was mucositis. The magic mouthwash wasn't a cure, but would help relieve the symptoms. Dr. Medica wasn't in favor of swallowing it when it contained lidocaine, but the modified version had a minimal amount of that analgesic, if any, so go ahead and drink the dose if it relieved my throat.

Better for keeping my mouth as healthy as possible was to swish frequently with baking soda and salt mixed in water. Twice as much baking soda as salt mixed in a cup of water in a container can be kept covered for days. Swish and spit it out.

I told her how I got laryngitis the first cycle. Dr. Medica's opinion was that the effect to my throat was caused by acid reflux—heartburn. She said you can have the silent type, where you don't feel symptoms. So now I had a prescription for Prilosec. One a day to keep the heartburn away—twice if I needed them.

The tics couldn't be helped, at least not by medication. In other words, be patient with my assaulted flesh.

My blood pressure was wacky: 151 over 58. (I never had bad blood pressure before being diagnosed with cancer; the doctor determined this was a consequence of the chemo. It could easily have gone the other direction and become low blood pressure.) She put me on a beta blocking blood pressure medication, Metoprolol, which works by relaxing blood vessels and slowing heart rate to improve blood flow and decrease blood pressure.

And because the head bone is connected to the hip bone, chemo was making my blood sugar (glucose) go up. The worst offender was probably Dexamethasone. It raises blood sugar levels, inducing Hyperglycemia. That was why I had frequent urination on Sunday night. Between Dexamethasone and the rich slice of chocolate cake that celebrated my fiftieth birthday (for the sixth time,) what did I expect? No, it was not diabetes; in fact I should resist taking a diabetes test for at least three months after chemo because I could have a false positive.

What are the effects of bad blood sugar? Damage to blood vessels and organs is a possibility. In untreated hyperglycemia, a condition called Ketoacidosis can occur. It develops when the body doesn't have enough insulin. Without insulin, the body isn't able to utilize glucose for fuel, so the body starts to break down fats for energy. It is a life-threatening condition which needs immediate treatment. Symptoms include shortness of breath, breath that smells fruity, nausea and vomiting, and very dry mouth.

Dr. Medica wanted me to modify my diet to keep my blood sugar down. Of course, the dietician wasn't in and I found confusing information on the Internet. I felt guilty that sugary grape juice had been my mainstay in the liquid department. It was the drink that tasted good enough to be drunk in volume when water tasted like dirt (hold the worms.) Someone suggested Perrier or another mineral water might be tolerable.

And they weren't going to let me slide. Dr. Sanatio's office called. I now had an appointment to get trained in taking insulin—probably not on a regular basis, hopefully not every day, just when I needed it. Tomorrow, remind me to ask about hypnosis for smoking as well. Might as well become a perfect person, if not perfectly healthy.

If I quit smoking, I wouldn't have any bad habits. So dull.

Friday, February 3, 2012

It felt like an eventful week. My legs had been achy, achy enough that I was not walking normally. Wednesday, I went to the doctor's office and got trained in giving myself insulin. I only cried twice. I had this awful feeling that I was destroying my health to save my life. Didn't want to do it. But I had to.

I had to go to Cottage Hospital to get the insulin supplies: the meter for measuring blood sugar, which included the sticker to poke my finger. In case you didn't know, the blood in the tip of the finger has the most accurate blood sugar count; you poke it with the special poker to make it bleed, stick the little paper strip into the meter, stick the paper strip on the blood, and see what the meter says.

Then, if you have to, you shoot yourself in the abdomen or thigh with a hypodermic needle of insulin. You can use a tiny little normal needle that you have to fill with the correct dose of insulin or use this honking big pen thing that is preloaded with insulin. With the pen, you dial a number to give the correct dose. I chose the pen because it was easier. I was into easy.

The insulin needle didn't hurt, which surprised me. I thought I would get a prick. Didn't feel the insulin either. I did feel the poke in the finger when I used the meter.

So, after I left Cottage Hospital, I stopped at the grocery store to get a couple of staple foods. Swiss cheese, crackers and for a treat, a small tray of shrimp. I was too tired to go to the pharmacy for the insulin. After she got home from work, Martha went to get it. One wasted trip. There was no prescription there.

Thursday, I was without a car. Slept till noon and felt incapable and useless until at least 3 pm. My guess is that I was dehydrated from not drinking while I overslept, plus needed calories to get my body up to speed. Munched shrimp, which almost tasted good, drank, and discovered that Perrier water, which tasted way too salty by itself, mixed well with regular water. It also went well in grape juice. You just need a splash to brighten up the flavors and dull the taste of mud.

My mouth was not that bad; I could taste things, but I couldn't get up the energy to make a phone call until late afternoon. Bad girl. Insulin was important, as I well knew, but I just couldn't do it. Finally, I called the doctor's office about the prescription. They were confused; it should have been with the papers that I took to Cottage Hospital.

I imitated a bump on a log for the rest of the day. At one point, I stood up and almost went right over on my back like a drunken turtle. That was a combination of my ears and the Prilosec, I believed. The Prilosec bottle warns it may cause dizziness.

Dependable, wonderful Rick fed me meatballs and bread and butter. He assured me the meatballs were delicious, as good as I ever made, but they didn't have flavor. The gravy did. There were two meatballs left; I would eat them tomorrow and gorge on the gravy. I went to bed feeling halfway decent. It took all day to get enough food and drink in me to gain equilibrium.

I woke at 5 am. My mouth was dry. I cursed myself for sleeping on my back and leaving my mouth hanging open, got up and made a cup of hot chocolate which did not relieve the dry mouth. Excuse my language, but oh, Hell. Now I had medical dry mouth, another side effect of chemo/ blood sugar. Or else I was just plain dehydrated.

Dry mouth is not the same as being thirsty. My lips, inside my mouth, even my throat were parched. Swallowing was a labor of Hercules. What spit was in my mouth made no difference. It's an infuriating sensation that you can't ignore. It makes you almost frantic to do something to relieve it.

Since I had to have the car to chase down insulin, I drove Martha to work, feeling miserable every mile. When I got home, I decided to have some bottled peaches; they should soothe my mouth, at least temporarily.

And they did. The dry mouth started to go away. (Maybe the sugar in the syrup did something. Don't know.)

I was very tired, but had enough energy to do what needed doing. I called the doctor's office and straightened out the snafu about the insulin prescription. They called it in to the pharmacy. I would have to drive up to get it. Also needed to put gas in the car. If I went to Janet's for food, that would expend the day's allowance of get up and go. But, if I was dehydrated, I should call the Breast Cancer clinic and see if I should come in for a bag of IV. Plump me up, make me feel good. Nah, not up to it. Let's wait another day. I retrieved the insulin. Never did get gas.

I had a serious lack of energy. Thank you, Mr. Cancer, for that.

Let's turn to vanity for a moment. I hadn't talked much about what chemotherapy did to my looks—to be honest, I am not very pretty and gave up a long time ago on looking great. I am average. I get blackheads on my nose, am overweight, and am very thankful my family loves me despite gray hair and idiosyncrasies.

Someone noticed the other day that I had no wrinkles. No, I didn't have a lot of them before, but I did have crow's feet and two vertical lines above my nose from squinting. They faded away. No doubt they would return, but a few months of no wrinkles was a smidge of compensation for having to go through chemo. I'll bet it was the fault of the steroids. They were making me look like a bulldog—I bet my skin was stretched. Well, if you have to have a misshapen head, you might as well be permanent press.

But last night, sitting in bed, having taken my vitamins and blood pressure pill like a good girl, I wiped my face with an Oil of Olay wipe. Then I made the mistake of grabbing the hand mirror to check my skin. When the chemo decides it is time to exit the body, where do you think it heads? For the pores, ma'am, for the pores (also out your urine, which is one reason to not dehydrate.) It seeps out and sits on your skin until you wipe or wash it off. The material from the Breast Cancer clinic indicates this starts about 72 hours after treatment. Last night was about 72 hours from Monday.

My poor face. The skin on my forehead peeled. It was like a chemical peel, only there wasn't a highly paid beautician picking off the dead stuff and bathing my forehead with a delicious smelling concoction guaranteed to give me smoother, younger looking skin. Instead, my forehead looked pitted, raw, unhappy. Rub a finger across the forehead and watch the skin fall on the bed. Ick.

I hadn't lost my eyebrows, though they were thinner than before chemo, especially the left one, but the skin under my brows needed sandblasting.

Then there was my nose. Every pore was huge and filled with blackheads. Gross, just plain gross. I gently scratched. Lo and behold, yellow, gnarly skin and blackheads came off with the scraping.

Doing what no medical personnel would ever advise, I spent the next half hour scraping my nose with my fingernails. Lightly, not enough to hurt, but enough to get the dead skin and blackheads off. My imagination said the black gunk was chemicals, but I didn't know. I just knew I couldn't stand to leave my nose alone. My tiny store of vanity had to get those blackheads off. I didn't have to squeeze, so I justified my actions. Scrape, wipe on Kleenex, and scrape again.

Once I cleaned my nose, it looked lumpy and the pores were still gigantic, but the blackheads were gone. So was the yellowish dead or dying skin. My skin felt irritated, but no more than if I had used a rough washcloth on it.

I surveyed my cheeks and gave up. No blackheads that I could see. Just two planes of extremely dry, lumpy, unhappy looking skin with white spots clogging enlarged pores. I needed a facial in the worst way. I went to sleep.

Today, my skin looked better. The pores were still enlarged, but not as big as last night. My nose looked clean, my cheeks wouldn't make babies cry, and my forehead was hanging in there. I am not sure what the doctors would advise—if getting a facial is a good idea or just more abuse to pile on top of abuse—but if you care what your skin looks like 72 hours after getting chemo, you might want to avoid mirrors. Just lightly scrub with a washcloth. Moisturize and deal with your skin when it isn't saturated with chemicals.

Saturday, February 4, 2012

The working world had the day off. I, who worked out of the house, didn't. How did people undergoing cancer treatment deal with work?

Some don't. They elect to stay home and fight cancer. Some want to work, but can't. Others continue to work full or part-time. They use up their vacation and sick time, take a leave of absence, start a medical leave, use short or long term disability insurance. Some leave their job to take a less demanding one. The options are limitless, provided their employer is understanding. Federal and state laws (The Family and Medical Leave Act and Americans with Disabilities Act for example,) might provide protection for your job. There might be provision for flex time, telecommuting, switching to a more flexible position. There might or might not be a paycheck. Or a full paycheck.

If you need or want to continue working while you go through the rigmarole of cancer treatment, talk to your employer, union rep, and doctors.

Plan to make adjustments in some way. Don't stubbornly insist on business as usual. Just know that, God willing, occupying a job can be done.

Sunday, February 5, 2012

Finally, I was starting to feel better. The vague feeling of malaise, as if I was thinking of getting the flu but not sure about it, eased up. It had been such a vague feeling I ignored it; only its absence made me recognize its existence. The muscles running down the inside of my thighs and down my calves stopped the restless aching that ibuprofen didn't touch. I even felt a bit of energy. Not a lot of energy, because I was not sleeping through the night, but a smidgen of interest in the world.

The coating on my tongue started to fall off. It was only on the back of my tongue, where it made swallowing unpleasant.

The next improvement should be in sleeping patterns. The last several days, I would sleep several hours, wake up, and be awake for four or five hours. Then I could fall back asleep and sleep a long time. Like till noon. I never sleep that late unless I am sick. Duh.

Last night, I just didn't get to sleep until late. Started to doze off, but then Bart the cat started picking on Tigerlily the cat and I had to go yell at Bart. That upset me, so I started to read. The light went off at 3 am. I was so brilliantly stupid; I had told Martha that I would go in for my blood test before she went to work so she could have the car. I had asked Rick to wake me up to make sure I went for my blood test before Martha went to work. Yes, I did as I said I would. I left at 7:45 am and was back by 8:30. Tired, feeling hung over, not energetic. Life can be a grind.

Yes, chemotherapy can cause insomnia. If the emotional issues involved with cancer don't keep you awake, if sleeping during the day doesn't keep you up at night, if side effects aren't disturbing your rest, if, if, if. The plain facts are that chemo disrupts the sleep-wake cycle.

A study showed that chemo patients were three times more likely to suffer insomnia than the general population. They think that emotional factors combine with something about the disease to create the problem. In other words, you and the cancer are working together to keep you awake.

Three quarters of the chemo patients in one study met the diagnostic criteria to be termed insomniac. Many of those people had problems sleeping throughout treatment. Those fighting breast cancer had the highest number of overall insomnia complaints. For the study, the syndrome was defined as difficulty sleeping three or more times a week for at least a month. Daytime tiredness and fatigue counted.

Insomnia can affect your immune system. It can bother your heart and become a chronic problem. You can ask the doctor to prescribe Ambien or another sleeping pill, but there are other things to try.

Providence Health & Services of Oregon & Southwest Washington has a list of products that might help you sleep better:

- Calms Forte, a homeopathic sleep aid, "is inexpensive and dead safe."
- Melatonin, a hormone involved with the sleep cycle, might help older folk. Start with a 3 mg dose 2-3 hours before bedtime, but do not use more than 20 mg. It might take a couple of days to kick in, so don't be discouraged if you don't immediately sleep like a baby.
- Valerian, a plant, has sedative effects. Get it in pill form and check that the label says "standardized extract"; you'll have a greater chance of it being a good quality herb. They recommend 600 mg one hour before bedtime as safe and effective. You can try less, but do not exceed 600 mg.
- Alcohol. Not usually something a doctor would advise, but a LITTLE nip of wine puts some people to sleep. If your sleep is disrupted, the small amount of alcohol you drink is probably outweighed by a good night's rest. Check with your doctor about this.
- A bedtime snack is not usually considered good for you, but if it helps you sleep, it helps you sleep.

Food in your tummy seems to have a calming effect. (For myself, as the list of drugs I had to take increased, I had to eat at bedtime to settle my stomach.) As the website advises, sip a cup of warm milk. Warm milk contains calcium, proteins and tryptophan, an essential amino acid that plays a role in relaxation and sleep. Some people make a hot milk nightcap by adding a quarter-shot of their favorite liqueur. Sprinkle nutritional yeast on popcorn; the yeast is rich in B vitamins and proteins, which also have a hand in drowsiness. Try peanut or almond butter on whole-grain bread, or a handful of almonds with a piece of fruit. The combination of carbohydrate and fat evens out the blood sugar. Cancer patients particularly benefit from a power yogurt sundae: plain yogurt high in beneficial bacteria mixed with high quality blueberry or raspberry jam and two tablespoons of ground flaxseed.

If you still can't sleep, don't beat yourself over the head. Lying in bed and staring at the ceiling isn't going to do much good. You'll just get all riled up over the fact that you can't get to sleep.

Get up and do something relaxing for 45 minutes and then go back to bed and try again. A good book is not relaxing, neither is a good movie. An extremely dull book or a TV show you would never willingly watch are better choices. Do something that doesn't rev up your body or mind. I found that I could fall asleep watching Martha's DVDs of The Big Bang Theory but NCIS kept me alert. With experimentation, you will find what activity and what length of time doing it is sufficient to put you to sleep.

You might discuss these products with your doctor before trying any of them. Your doctor might suggest something else. Don't ignore insomnia; you don't want it to become a habit.

The side effect I was most peeved at lately was the sensitivity of my fingernails. They had been almost sore for nearly a week. I was typing with the balls of my fingers, trying to avoid my nails. I couldn't open a pop top can. My fear was that this was the harbinger of my nails falling off, but who knows? The thumbs were dark near the cuticle, but not nearly as dark as pictures on the Internet show can happen. A couple of other nails were darkening, but the thumbs were the worst. The affected nails humped like spoons and the thumbs had a couple of deep ridges going across them.

The index finger on my left hand developed overnight a white line going across that looked like a bit of cuticle stuck on the nail. This is called Beau's lines and although it doesn't look pretty, it is harmless. As the nails grow out, you can trim the lines off. The nerves in my hand didn't go numb, or twitch, or do anything upsetting this chemo cycle, so I didn't have any basis to believe my fingernails were going to dry up and blow away. It was an irrational fear.

Actually, the Internet says that any and all damage done to the nails by chemo is temporary. It will all disappear after chemotherapy as the nails grow out. Growing an entire nail from cuticle to tip can take six months or more, so patience is a virtue.

Just be nice to your nails. They don't like a lot of water and soap but they do appreciate moisturizer. Leave the cuticles alone so they don't tear; pushing the cuticle back is not best practice. If the skin along the sides gets uber dry, as mine did, you can go so far as to soak your fingers in warm cooking oil to help soften things up. Rub the oil in; it will coat the nails and help with brittleness. Keeping them shorter and squaring the nails rather than rounding them will give them the best chance of remaining strong.

My nails seemed thick. This might have been because I wasn't cleaning under them with a nail file; they were just too sensitive to bother. Then again, it really looked like the nails were thicker. Concerted cleaning with the file (another finger holding the nail down so I didn't push it off) took a lot of work and the underside didn't clean evenly. I gave up. "Let them grow out and work on them later," I said to myself. Little did I realize it was the nails growing wrongly due to chemicals. It would fix itself.

Remember, during chemo you are more prone to infection and that includes around nails.

My skin, on the other hand, had already dried up and blown away. A bottle of Vaseline Intensive Care wouldn't make a dent in the desert that was my forearms. My palms were turning white with dryness. Did you know I detest the feel of moisturizer?

And I thought my chest port shifted more. It was uncomfortable; the spot in my neck where the port threaded through the vein pinched. Maybe I should call the Breast Cancer clinic and get it checked, but I was pretty sure they weren't going to do anything. They were going to tell me not to worry about it. They wouldn't touch it unless they couldn't access it, and they wouldn't try until my next chemo treatment.

I think lack of sleep was making me paranoid. I took a nap after Bart the cat settled down.

Tuesday, February 7, 2012

La di da, a decent day. I had become comfortable testing my blood sugar and shooting up with insulin. It helped that I invariably needed the lowest dose. Made me feel less like a diabetic and more like a chemo patient with a nasty side effect. Don't tell me that I had been assured that I was not diabetic. Emotions don't listen to reason.

The diabetes supplies were piled in one plastic basket that I could carry wherever they were needed. Most common was in front of the computer and in front of the TV. I was supposed to test morning, afternoon and night, either before, during or after eating. I was sleeping all morning, so I tested around noon, about five, and after my evening ice cream.

Oh, yes, I still enjoyed my evening chocolate ice cream. With Dr. Sanatio's permission, I may add. Actually, I didn't have ice cream for nearly a week and that was when I seemed to have more problems with dehydration. I could justify that ice cream. It was a highly pleasurable way to get liquid down my gullet and I cried real tears, right there in his office, when Dr. Sanatio said I shouldn't have it.

Since my appetite had fallen off, ice cream was more important than ever. Satisfying my stomach had become a priority. I did try for good nutrition, but if something settled well and made an attempt to taste good, I had trouble resisting it. One of the things the experts say is "If you can't eat well, eat what you can."

I remembered that the doctor said that chemo tended to make people hungrier, but you couldn't prove it with me, certainly not these last several days. My interest in food and drink dropped measurably after I began taking insulin, perfectly normal, according to the Internet. Insulin makes you less hungry. I wanted an Oreo, but there weren't any in the house. I would survive without Oreos, but I had to have my ice cream.

I reviewed the lists of side effects of chemo and thought I had escaped one. Chemo brain. Caused (they think) by nerve damage in the brain, chemo brain is a lot like menopause—you go vague, can't remember things, drive everyone crazy. Nope, I wasn't doing that. All the craziness I could throw at Martha was caused by the normal things I do that make her crazy.

People were starting to ask how I was doing on chemo. Was it working? I didn't have any idea. That constituted the one and only question I had for the doctor.

I believed my hair was growing. When I walked, I could feel this soft down drifting around my head. Hats were as bad as they ever were. The only two I wanted to wear were knitted winter hats; the red one Martha bought me lived on my bed, ready to wear when needed. When I went out in public, I wore the black skull cap from the American Cancer Society tlc catalog. With modification to the elastic, it was no longer too tight, and with a gauzy headband that coordinated with my chemo shirts, it looked ok. But it tended to slide up like it was going to pop off. I decided my neck was too short for hats. Tilt my head and my neck pushed the hat up.

My nose was runnier than usual, though this would be hard to prove without catching it all in a cup and measuring. For sure not going to do that. I only noticed it because someone in a cancer chat room mentioned it.

If my nose was runnier, I bet I knew the reason. Chemo drugs are trained to attack cancer cells which grow like madmen, but aren't smart enough to know to leave perfectly nice fast growing cells alone. The drugs go after mucus membranes as well as cancer cells because mucus membranes renew themselves faster than, for example, bones. Mucus membranes are up the nose, around the mouth, wherever you get damp from the inside. My poor assaulted mucus membranes were crying after being beat up.

Except for consistent diarrhea, I was good to go until the next chemo treatment. I hoped.

Friday, February 10, 2012

My blood sugar was dropping toward normal levels. The first day I tested, I had to give myself three injections. Two of those injections were the minimum dose, but one was the next higher dose. Today I had to give myself only one injection. Makes sense, if the insulin problem was caused by the steroids. The longer you go after taking the steroids (which was Dexamethasone the day before, the day of, and the day after the chemo treatment) the less influence they would have on the body. Cross your fingers that I could stop doing insulin by next week. Then I would have a whole week free of poking myself.

As a pretend diabetic, I noticed the amount of sugar I ate, all while I was trying to stick to a more healthy diet. I was not drinking soda pop because it didn't taste good. I had switched to bottled water splashed with Perrier and fruit juice. I was doing okay with purple grape, low acid orange, and apple. I found that strawberry peach was pretty good. Have you read the nutrition labels on juice? They have an awful lot of sugar in them. When the label says "juice from concentrate" there is even more sugar. My nightly chocolate ice cream was also loaded. If I was really diabetic, I couldn't have them.

Loads of carbohydrates are a no no for diabetics; too many carbs shoots blood sugar up. My husband's preference for pasta or potato dinners nagged at my "diabetic" brain. I did learn on the Internet that someone tested different foods and found that the parts of potatoes, rice, and maybe pasta that upset glucose tend to change if the foods are leftovers. So cooking them, throwing them in the fridge, and reheating them when you want to eat them may help. Also from the Internet, I picked up the idea that our bodies are wired to have problems with insulin; we make extra insulin at the drop of a hat, but don't have an easy way to get rid of too much. It is ironic that having problems with insulin are "cured" by taking more insulin.

Diet is incredibly important to the topic. The best diet comes with the best lifestyle. For diabetics, the ideal lifestyle is that of a cave man. Great. I'll live in a cave, eating roots, leaves, the occasional berry and the even more occasional tyrannosaurus rex. Since the tyrannosaurus rex is more likely to eat me, I won't live long and won't have to worry about diabetes. The human race needs a medical breakthrough on the treatment of this disease.

One side effect I missed was hot flashes and/or night sweats. I had one episode during Cycle 1. If you went through menopause or lived with a woman who did, you probably know what they are: sudden heat that makes you sweat and swear often followed by chills.

What do you do about it? Wear cotton—it will absorb sweat better than other materials. Wear layers so you can add or remove them as necessary. Keep a fan available; avoid warm, stuffy rooms. Limit spicy foods, large meals and sugar. Caffeine encourages the heat, as does alcohol. Drink plenty of healthy fluids to avoid dehydration. Vitamin E, selenium and

B6 seem to help, but check with the doctor before popping supplements. According to studies, soy products don't do much good, although positive claims are made for them. A couple of companies make wipes that soothe the skin; blue packaged Olay is one I am familiar with. Try to find one that isn't perfumed and is alcohol free.

Turning beet red and sweating like a pig is not comfortable or socially desirable, but if it is a cost of surviving cancer, you can grin and bear it.

Tuesday, February 14, 2012

Happy Valentine's Day. I was not doing anything special; I didn't have the car, it was snowy and cold, and most of our disposable income should go to Henry Ford Health System. What I would do was cook Rick a wonderful meal. I had a roast in the freezer and potatoes in the cupboard. Martha and Katie would get loving emails. I'd get a nap. That would cover Valentine's Day.

I was perturbed about my blood sugar readings. They hovered just above the minimum and every once in a while they shot up. They did not go to normal. So I cruised the Internet looking for something that would tell me how long the steroids that elevate blood sugar levels stay in the body. The only sites that gave usable information dealt with studies done on administering Dexamethasone before surgery. In those studies, the patients were followed for about four hours. What happens if you take the steroid for three days every three weeks? If you were sensitive to steroids? I would have to ask the oncologist.

The issue I had with steroids dated back to treatment of my sinus infections. For several years I had a prescription for Nasacort, a steroid spray that opens up the sinuses. It worked well; I sprayed Nasacort into my nose, using less than the prescribed dose, and was able to breathe fairly well. After I had surgery to straighten the septum in my nose, the surgeon said I could use Nasacort up to four times a day with no ill effects. I sprayed and sprayed, and then the eye doctor told me I had glaucoma.

It turns out that the steroid in Nasacort causes glaucoma (high pressure in the eyes which can damage vision and even cause blindness) in something like a quarter of the people who use it. Nasacort can also cause cataracts. Yep, I got cataracts also, but they weren't bad enough to do anything about. I stopped using Nasacort and over the course of a year, my eye pressure came down to high normal. Judging from the results of a small study I found on the Internet, I had hopes that another six months sans steroids would cure my glaucoma, the idea being that the pressure was caused by Nasacort, not by my body malfunctioning.

Though skeptical of the study, Dr. Eye Doctor said I might be a steroid responder; I might be extra sensitive to steroids and their side effects. I resolved never to use steroids again unless absolutely necessary. Going blind is a worst case scenario to me, the lady who loves to read, enjoys computer games, and has done needlepoint as a much loved hobby for more than forty years. If you don't know what needlepoint is, it is related to embroidery. Blind people can't needlepoint. I'd rather be in a wheelchair than blind.

So there I was, triple negative breast cancer fighter, using steroids that raised my blood pressure and blood sugar. My eyesight was getting worse—the eye doctor warned me it would. He said it would actually be good if the breast cancer treatments made the cataracts worse because then we could do something about them.

Yes, chemo drugs can make cataracts. They can also cause dry eye syndrome, watery eyes, itchy eyes, and other problems. Check with an eye doctor (ophthalmologist) during chemo to be aware of incoming trouble.

I needed to visit the eye doctor and have him check the glaucoma and cataracts. And I needed to explore the blood sugar and blood pressure issue more. Could the steroid make me truly diabetic or give me permanently high blood pressure? What kind of pit was I digging? I wanted to be warned.

Random facts

- The left breast is statistically more prone to developing cancer than the right breast. Scientists are unsure why.
- When breast cancer shows up on that blasted mammogram, it may have been in your body for 6-10 years.
- Researchers discovered tell-tale signs of cancer in a 3,000 year old skeleton. Did they use hemlock for chemo?

Friday, February 17, 2012

I don't know if it is the chemo or something else, but I blame you, Cancer, for the shortness of breath and weakness in my legs the last two days. It came on suddenly. Tuesday night I felt fine. Wednesday was awful. Did it make you giggle to see me so messed up?

Damn you, Cancer. No matter what you throw at me, I will make do, get around, climb over. And I will kick you. So stay out of my way. Get out of my life.

Weakness is a common occurrence in cancer fighters. It is not the same as tiredness, it is feeling unable physically. Chemo drugs mess with muscles and the muscles weaken. According to an Internet chat room, one man was so weak he had to crawl up stairs. It can be that debilitating. In this situation, more exercise does not equal improvement. People who were athletes before chemo became weak as well as more sedentary folk like me, who spend hours on the computer.

What was up with my legs? I couldn't tell until I discussed it with the oncologist, but I could describe symptoms. It began in the long muscles in the front of my thighs. They felt weak, tired. By the time I walked halfway to the store, a matter of at most 150 feet, my thighs were trembling. The muscles in my calves were next; they began to knot up and feel tired. Weak. Breathing was bad, but not bad enough to make me dizzy.

The people at the store know me well. They were fine with me leaning against the counter, taking some of the pressure off my legs, until I felt well enough to walk home. My legs were sooooo tired when I got home and I was somewhat unsteady on my feet.

I rested and looked for clues on the Internet. That was how I heard about the man crawling up stairs. No one knows what is going on with the muscles weakening. Some sites claim it is a form of neuropathy, some class it as its own symptom—weakness. One site hinted that it might be a matter of the muscles failing to slide properly in their sheaths.

I didn't know muscles have sheaths. They are supposed to be called fascia. Wikipedia says, "Fasciae are similar to ligaments and tendons as they are all made of collagen except that ligaments join one bone to another bone, tendons join muscle to bone and fasciae connect muscles to other muscles." The suggestion was that massage might help correct badly sliding muscles. So I banged my thighs with my fists and then asked Rick to massage my legs.

Rick's massage revealed that the muscles in my thighs had knotted up as much as those in my calves. Rubbing them was painful, but in the good massage painful way. Unfortunately, The University of Maryland Medical Center says that massage is not recommended for chemotherapy patients as it can damage tissue made frail by chemo drugs, so I shouldn't have Rick beat up my legs unless and until the doctor said he could do it.

That night, I took a Naproxen, which functions as a muscle relaxant for me. Thursday, I was more mobile, although my legs still felt weak.

So I would stretch and exercise my legs more. Monday, when I went for my 4th chemo treatment, I would discuss weakness and breathing with Dr. Medica.

The hair under my left arm (the side where the lymph nodes were removed) was growing better than under my right arm, meaning I could see a couple tiny little hairs. I lost a few more hairs from my eyebrows, especially from the outsides, but they did not look deformed. I had a basic number of eyelashes, nowhere near enough for Cover Girl to ask me to film an ad.

I think the hair on my head was growing. If so, it looked to be more dark than gray, but you couldn't really tell. I had some hair on my legs (never lost it all) but it was negligible. Baby hair. The hairs that had developed on my face after menopause—I suffered the incipient Bearded Lady of the circus that makes lots of women buy all those hair loss products—well, some of them were coming back, darn it. Pubic hair was sparse to nonexistent. Nope, no hair on my toes. Just out of curiosity, I checked. Hair on toes was not a big deal ever. Not much on my arms and what was there was light colored and wispy.

I can't say I liked the state of my head, but around the house, I didn't pay attention to it. Rick and Martha got used to the way I looked. When Rick and I went to the grocery store, I wanted to take the hat off because I was hot. The thought of scaring children kept it on.

Reminding myself that I'd had only two or three outbreaks of hemorrhoids lately, I wrote Cottonelle wipes on the grocery list. I still had loose stools, but not so much diarrhea. My urine was bright lemon yellow—it was too concentrated, so I assumed I was fighting dehydration, but the color was off. Was it drugs coming out of my system?

Sunday, February 19, 2012

The big toe environs of both of my feet were a little numb today. That was neuropathy, pure and simple. My hands felt fine. Tics around my eyes continued ad nauseum.

My blood sugar was 156 when I checked it at breakfast. Then, at lunch, it was 278, and after dinner 332, the highest it had been. Scared me, made me mad, and then I remembered that I took two Dexamethasone pills today as required for the chemo treatment tomorrow. It was Dexamethasone they blamed for my screwy blood sugar levels. If I had any doubts, they were wiped away.

I would have Dexamethasone in the IV tomorrow. Tuesday I had to take two more pills. It was firmly in my mind that if my blood sugar went above 500 I was to call. Not going to forget that.

Chemotherapy Cycle 4

Tuesday, February 21, 2012

Yesterday was chemo. Martha worked from home, so getting to the hospital by 9 am was no hassle. I had some leg weakness; getting from the car to the 13th floor of Henry Ford Hospital was an effort. I was weighed—standing steady about five pounds down, which was a grin. I couldn't remember the last time I managed to lose five pounds, much less keep it off.

I had blood drawn. Despite the tipping of the chest port, the nurse had no difficulty accessing it. That was one worry relieved. If the port stopped working, they would have to take it out and probably put one in my arm. That would delay treatment.

We saw Dr. Medica. She likes Godiva and Nestles, but not Hershey's. I'm not so particular. I should buy her some Godiva—she deserved it because she got a genuine smile on her face when she saw me. I asked my questions.

How could we tell if the chemo was working? Surprisingly, Dr. Medica said that we didn't have any way of knowing if it was doing anything. My treatment was based on what has been done in the past that seemed to work plus studies (AKA clinical trials) done in the field.

In other words, with all the people treated for breast cancer in the past, doctors have learned what seems to work well and what doesn't pan out. Studies eliminated some ideas as being not so great, but suggested others worth pursuing. Comparing my tumors with those of past cancer fighters and the good things studies came up with, they chose the treatment plan for me that produces the best results.

It's a creepy guessing game, but at least it is an informed guessing game. We would know how well it worked for me if and when I didn't grow more cancer.

How long does Dexamethasone stay in the body? Dr. Medica couldn't remember the exact length of time, but she was pretty sure it would be gone in 4 days. She offered to check, but I said it didn't matter. Since I was concerned about my blood sugar count, I asked to talk to the dietician to see what I should eat to help even things out.

The dry mouth I suffered was caused by blood sugar. She reminded me to swish with the baking soda/salt/water solution and suggested I get an over-the-counter preparation, Biotine, to coat my mouth. It eases the unpleasant feeling caused by the dryness and protects the mouth from damage.

Yes, the mouth, including teeth, can be harmed by dryness. I searched the Internet to see what others recommend. Everyone mentioned Biotine. Other measures that are helpful are sipping water frequently, sucking hard candies to produce saliva (watch the sugar,) use lip moisturizer, and use a cool mist humidifier at night. By the way, Biotine comes in toothpaste, mouth spray, liquid, oral rinse, gum, and gel. Sounded like they covered every way a person might want to use it.

I reported the numbness in my toes and weakness in my legs. It's all neuropathy. When my legs were troublesome, avoid sitting for long periods. Walk around for five minutes, but don't overdo it. The idea was to keep blood flowing, not to wear myself out. If my legs got bad enough, they would delay chemo to give them time to recover. She didn't want me to become disabled from it. Ditto for breathing.

I told her treatment was the highest priority; I would dislike delaying chemo. We left it at that.

My urine was lemon colored. Dr. Medica thought it must be something I was eating. Couldn't imagine what unless it was the strawberry peach fruit drink, but I didn't drink any last night and still was lemony. (After the fact, and with no proof, it may have been caused by a steady diet of vitamins.)

She checked my lymph nodes and left breast and then Rick and I were free until 11, when chemo was scheduled. We went outside for a cigarette, a long walk that taxed me. That was the first time it dawned on Rick that I was serious about weakness in my legs, but he didn't comment. He just patiently waited while I took a break on a bench.

It had been a quick visit with the oncologist, so we had time to eat breakfast in the cafeteria—if it wasn't closed from 10-10:30 for them to switch from the breakfast to lunch menu. So we got muffins and a banana from the coffee shop and ate light. Then I insisted on another cigarette; mentally preparing myself for chemo wasn't easy and if I wanted to smoke, I wanted to smoke. After, we went up to the waiting room. Only twenty minutes until I would be called in. It went fast.

I was hooked up to the IV when the dietician showed up. She had the American Diabetes Association's guidelines by heart. I should count carbohydrates. Carbs are what push blood sugar up; simple carbs (foods like chocolate, most packaged cereal, and potato chips) send blood sugar skyrocketing right away, but more complex carbs (most beans, cheese, strawberries—but no strawberries during chemo) take longer to get it moving. I should aim for 60 grams of carbs per meal. How I got them was my choice. There are lists on the Internet (search for "counting carbs" to turn up oodles) and see how you like the idea of this diet. 60 grams of carbohydrates isn't a meal. Of course I could add any amount of protein to fill me up.

Chemo went fast. The nurse must have been efficient; we were done fifteen minutes early.

That night, we wanted Paczki (pronounce it punchkie and you will get by,) the extra rich jelly donuts the Polish eat on Fat Tuesday (the day before Lent starts.) I am half Polish, but my family never indulged. We didn't "do" Lent either and the Easter Bunny was more important than Jesus. Anyway, Martha went to the store and came back with Paczki. We ate stew, then I had two cream cheese filled Paczki. Want to guess my blood sugar levels?

In the morning, after a banana, a blueberry muffin and apple juice, I tested at 234. At lunch, 279, then I ate a grilled corned beef sandwich with Swiss cheese on rye and splurged on a Coke. At dinner, 285, followed by beef stew, water and carb loaded Paczki. The next morning, my blood sugar was 195.

Normal levels are around 150 after dinner and under 120 in the am. Do you see why I had this niggling feeling that food was not determining my levels? One of these days, when the Dexamethasone was out of my system, I should follow the Atkins diet (all protein) and see what my sugar tested at.

A note about steroids: Steroids are powerful drugs. They do wondrous things, but can also mess up the body royally. If you are a steroid responder (sensitive to the drugs) the effects can be doubled or tripled. What gets me is that oncologists use steroids to protect the chemoed body from excessive harm, but seem to be careless about their adverse effects. If Dexamethasone commonly raises blood sugar in chemo patients, why didn't I find any studies about it? I found precious little info about steroid induced diabetes on the Internet. Is it a conspiracy?

No, there's no conspiracy. There just doesn't seem to be a lot of interest in the subject. Diabetes is accepted as an unfortunate but unavoidable side effect of steroid use in chemotherapy. My guess is that oncologists accept this because there isn't any alternative. Steroids do enough good that the bad has to be accepted. You would think someone would want to see if they could find a solution. All I knew was that steroids seemed to be hanging around in my system for an extended time, raising Cain.

Katie would fly in tonight from Sacramento. I needed to take a nap and then clean the bathroom. Maybe I'd get in some other cleaning also, but the bathroom was the priority. That and the bedroom she would use. And the kitchen... and the living room... forget floors. Someone else would have to vacuum carpets and wash down wood floors. Bart, the long haired cat, was shedding white clumps all over the green carpet.

Before cleaning, I went to the Cancer Genetics Clinic to find out the results of my testing. Thanks to the wonder of paper, I now knew the geneticist's name: Dr. Scientia. Somehow, I screwed up the time. I was there at 7:45 and my appointment was at 11. Dr. Scientia wiggled around and saw me anyway. Thank you not only for messing with your schedule to accommodate me, but for the results. Negative all the way around.

They didn't find any sign of mutations, BRCA or otherwise. There could be something that science was not aware of, but I didn't have to worry about Dr. Medica wanting to schedule a double mastectomy. More importantly, it eased fears that I had passed a ticking time bomb to my daughters.

They had a sample letter on the Internet that I could send to my family. I preferred a simple email.

And so far, very few side effects from yesterday's chemo. Water didn't taste good, but it was tolerable. Not a lot of energy, but I was up at 5:30 am, exceptionally early, went to the Cancer Genetics Clinic, delivered a laptop, ate at Janet's, stopped at the store and bought Cheerios for Katie, and wrote. Surprise, surprise, no house cleaning got done.

It was time for a nap.

Friday, February 24, 2012

Katie is here! What a relief. Blessing. Godsend. I wanted both of my babies near me and for a week, they were. It added emotional security to an unsettled time. In other words, it made me feel GOOD.

She didn't mind that I hadn't cleaned for her arrival. She just did it herself. She also cleaned the back stairs, shuffled the pile of donations out of the basement and to the Salvation Army, took me to the eye doctor, and worked on our taxes.

Our taxes were a mess. Between Rick's job, my two jobs as writer and computer consultant, and the rental income from our duplex, there was a lot involved and I failed to organize things this year.

The most important thing she did was hug me.

While Katie was Superwoman, saving me from myself, I quietly suffered. I was constipated Tuesday. That resolved itself Wednesday, but my stomach was more sensitive this cycle. Still no throwing up but nourishment went to the bottom of the list of important things. Boo, hiss.

I decided that effects to the mouth are the worst part of chemo. Dry mouth again this morning, relieved by drinking a whole glass of strawberry peach juice in one fell swoop. Strawberry peach tasted like straight sugar, so I switched back to good old grape. Hard boiled eggs were dreadful.

Everything tasted like dirt, even chocolate. Well, chocolate was not quite that bad, but it didn't taste good. I don't know if I didn't suck enough ice when the IVs started or if it was just the luck of the draw, but I was not looking forward to eating and drinking this week. The roof of my mouth felt slimy. Yep, what chemo does to your mouth is the pits.

I had a good report from the eye doctor. The glaucoma was holding steady and my tear ducts were not being ruined by the drugs. Remember, if you don't rinse the chemo drugs out of your eyes on a regular basis, they can permanently narrow the tear ducts. Not happening here. He gave me a bunch of samples for different versions of Refresh eye drops so I could drown my eyes.

I was going to lose the last of my eyelashes soon and he didn't think the twitches around my lids were significant. The steroids were making my face rounder; the technician stretched my glasses so they were not so tight over my ears. Wish she could stretch my clothes as well. I had not gained weight, but the fat was rearranging itself—not in a good way. When does something good happen?

Katie is good. Martha is good. Rick is good. So are the cats. I didn't need anything else.

My fingernails continued to darken and they were sensitive again. I needed to cut them short so I could type. I could feel neuropathy in my right hand (minimal,) both feet (minimal to tolerable,) and my thighs and arms around the elbows felt sorry for themselves. I was tired most of the time.

Sadly, I wasn't wholly aware of Katie's presence as the days went by. I completely missed when she went to the art museum for the afternoon. I was too wrapped in misery to fully appreciate my little family in one big piece in our little house. How much do you enjoy a loved one's presence when you are lolling around sick with the flu? How talkative are you when you are hit with pneumonia?

Had to go through this two more times. I was over the hump—I had completed three chemo cycles and was into the fourth—but the emotional rush did not last. It was a drag, thinking about having to do the whole thing two more times. If I had normal cancer, not triple negative, I would be at the end of chemo.

Saturday, February 25, 2012

Rick and Martha went to look at used cars. When I started radiation therapy, I would need a car every day and she was going to need one as the re-election campaign for the congressman heated up. Just didn't ask where the money was going to come from. I supposed I would squeak it out of somewhere, as usual. I'm a financial wizard with a bare bones budget.

The mud effect in my mouth was replaced by a salt lick. I could taste salt all the time, even when I ate chocolate. I checked with the doctor's office; the salt lick was classified with the general side effect of altered taste.

Katie served me a slice of ham and a bowl of applesauce for lunch. My tongue was coated; with the resultant lack of taste, ham and applesauce were a good choice to soothe my mouth. Finished eating, read a good book, and wham, the gods struck me down.

Out of the blue, a volcano of acid rose out of my stomach, flowing straight up into my mouth. No bile, no solid anything, just pure acid. At least the citizens of Pompeii had warning before they were killed by Vesuvius; I had nothing to suggest doom.

With Katie hovering, I tried to figure out what to do. I was not well-versed in heartburn or acid reflux; this was nothing like the very occasional heartburn I had suffered in my life. A long, protracted drink of water did nothing. A call to the doctor's office was not answered. Saturday, don't you know.

The pharmacist informed me that an additional dose of Omeprazole, the generic Prilosec sitting in front of me on the desk, would not save me. Katie ran to the corner store and got some Tum Tum Tum Tum Tums. Within half an hour I had taken double the recommended dose and could almost relax. My voice faded to a squeak, the corners of my mouth were burned. The inside of my mouth felt like it had been bathed in acid, which it had. My sternum (breastbone) felt weird, kind of numb.

Rick, our resident acid reflux expert, said it was probably a mixture of the salt in the ham and the acid in the applesauce that brought me low.

I ate ham and applesauce regularly during the first chemo cycle with no problem but I might never eat them again. Taking Rick's advice, I switched to Martha's bottle of Pepcid, took one before bedtime along with my generic Prilosec, and slept propped up so the contents of my stomach would not be encouraged to backflow up my throat.

What should you do about heartburn, or acid reflux, or whatever you want to call it? WebMD says to avoid the foods that bring the acid on, eat smaller meals more frequently, don't eat at least two to three hours before lying down, don't wear tight clothing or belts, try sleeping more upright. Also limit caffeine and fatty foods. I could add "Skip Chemo."

Products like Alka-Seltzer, Maalox, Mylanta, Rolaids, Tums, Pepcid or Zantac help neutralize the acid. If you take too many pills you risk constipation or diarrhea, surely an acceptable risk when you think you are going to die. Less acceptable is that taking too many can encourage C Diff (read in the Radiology chapter to learn about C Diff.)

Omeprazole let me down. A proton-pump inhibitor, it is supposed to suppress gastric acid secretions by inhibiting the enzyme pump process, which is the final step in the production of gastric acid secretions. It didn't.

I suggest you buy a bottle of whatever and have it on hand. If you don't need it, great. If you do need it, you need it NOW.

Sunday, February 26, 2012

My stomach settled. The coating on my tongue was giving up the ghost. Maybe I was pulling out of side effect season.

I was no longer going out except for necessities like blood tests. Someone else went to the grocery store and the pharmacy. I'd like to say I was being prudent, avoiding sources of infection, but the sorry truth was I didn't feel good enough to go out. I didn't pay attention to the rest of the world, either.

It was becoming clear that the Bashara murder was solved; the husband killed the wife. That news floated into my head, since I had vaguely known the couple, but little else did. I was in a fog most of the time. When Katie went back to Sacramento, I cried and felt worse.

Sunday, March 4, 2012

Dear Cancer,
I'm tired of whining. How about a change of pace? I'll list some of the things I have to be happy about.

Lying in bed the other night, I decided I qualify as a cancer survivor. No, I don't know that I have beaten you yet, stinky old Mr. Cancer, but I am fighting as best I can. I deserve a blue ribbon with the words "Cancer Survivor" emblazoned in gold leaf. I don't feel incredibly bad while I am fighting you, either. Yes, there are aches and pains, plenty of inconveniences, and twinges of real discomfort, but nothing I can't live with. I repeat: I can live with it.

I have a supportive family. They listen to me whine. They smile when I am bitchy. They love me when I am impossible. And they put up with me falling asleep four times in one evening while Martha researched the purchase of her car. After my concern about financing, she was handling it herself. I guess my baby had grown up. I missed the discussion, but I'd get to ride in her newly leased Ford Focus when it arrived. I approved of her color choice.

That's an old family joke. When I bought my first new car, I did almost as well as Martha, investigating what was available, what I could afford, what I liked. When I walked into the dealership, I knew exactly what I wanted. The only thing I didn't know was what color they had available. The salesman thought that was all I cared about. Life lesson: don't make snap judgments. I won't assume that salesman was an ass if he won't decide I was an airhead.

I had made progress on my genealogy. No, I hadn't found Joseph Keeler, but I was making headway with the French family in Buckinghamshire, England. That was personal satisfaction.

My house was cleaner, thanks to Katie. Don't fault Martha; she was working 10-12 hour days and couldn't keep up with me, the house, and the congressman. Dust would move in unless I found the energy to bustle around, but who cares? The sun was shining, it was supposed to be almost 60° outside by the end of the week, and in the Midwest, that is something to celebrate. Winter was losing grip. We would be able to go out without muffling to the ears.

The cats cuddled with me when I slept. Since I slept a lot, they were getting lots of cuddles.

There is plenty to be thankful for. And I am thankful to be able to enjoy my blessings.

Here's me sticking my tongue out at you, Cancer.

Monday, March 5, 2012

Back to business. You didn't buy this book to read maudlin fancies. You want to know what to watch for going through the grim business of fighting breast cancer. So let's deal with realities—just don't forget your blessings.

Rick said I had been overreacting to everything. I didn't see it, but we assumed it was a result of the chemo. I did the same thing during menopause. Should be temporary—it had better be temporary! I would try not to do it.

The baby toe on my left foot had been sensitive for several days. I stuck it in Martha's face and asked if she could see anything. Yep, it was not happy. Some of the toenails were turning dark to match the fingernails. The left baby toenail, while not really black, looked like it was losing its mooring. Yucko if it decided to fall off. Talking to a friend who was on the track team in high school, I knew that toenails falling off is not the end of the world. Runners lose theirs to the constant friction of running shoes. Grin and bear it. The fingernails were sensitive, but didn't feel loose.

The sole of my left foot peeled. I took a rough washcloth to both of my feet, scrubbing dead skin off. The right foot was hardly worth doing; it was the left that shed a whole layer. My forehead was spared this time. It flaked, but didn't outright peel.

The peeling on my foot may have been a mild case of Hand-Foot Syndrome or Palmar-Plantar Erythrodysesthesia, a condition where small amounts of chemo drugs leak out of capillaries in the palms of the hands and soles of the feet. It causes tenderness, redness, and sometimes peeling of the skin. It can be bothersome enough that chemo has to be interrupted. To counter the problem, you have to reduce friction (lots less walking,) limit exposure to heat (no hot baths,) and avoid rubbing the skin (no lotions) for a week after chemo sessions. Vitamin B6 might help in prevention and treatment. Me? I dodged the bullet. I did have some redness and the skin peeled, but I had no pain.

The biggie was now my thigh muscles. They felt weak. Sometimes walking was hard; other times, it was surprisingly possible. Problems breathing went along with the weakness in my legs. If my legs were bad, I had difficulty breathing. Trouble catching my breath. Just plain out of breath. I had to use a cane to help me walk at least some of the time.

Feeling great trepidation, I went to the grocery store with Rick. Getting down the front steps and to the car was chancy. The trip from the house to the car was tiring; I fell into the car seat rather than seating myself. "I am a fool," I thought. "I should send Rick to the store and stay home." But I wanted out of the house, the shopping list was in my head, not on paper, and Rick is notorious for impulse buying.

My fear was that I wouldn't make it through the store; going up and down aisles, backtracking for mushrooms from the produce department when I decided in the meat section that stew was a good idea. Hence Rick's presence. He could backtrack, as long as I was strict about impulse purchases. I could stand at the top of an aisle and send him down it for mayo. Sure, I could have used the motorized shopping cart, but I would be damned before I did that.

I "drove" the cart, which meant I could lean on it. I made it through produce, bread, soup and mayo. I got to the meat department before my thighs got really tired. Grrrr. Then my legs surprised me. Yes, they were tired, yes, they ached, but they didn't give out. By the time we got back to the car, I was walking slowly, but I was still walking. Victory.

When we got home, I collapsed into a chair and let Rick and Martha put the groceries away.

One purchase was two pounds of hamburger. I would make patties, fry them, and put cheese on top. Hamburgers without buns. I craved protein. The salt lick in my mouth had eased; I didn't taste it as much. Ground beef and cheese were an okay protein pairing. Unfortunately, I quickly lost my taste for cheese covered hamburger patties.

Neuropathy may be a pain, but blood clots are a side effect I escaped. Their formation during chemo is more likely because the components of the blood are messed up. A clot, which is nothing more or less than a thickened jelly-like mass of blood, becomes dangerous when it manages to block the flow of blood through a vein or artery.

These be dangerous waters, matie. Watch for pain, swelling, discoloration, or prominent veins in the leg, which can indicate a clot down there. If a clot is in the head, symptoms include numbness or weakness, often on one side of the body, or sudden severe headache, confusion, balance problems—any or all of the things you think of as part of a stroke. If a clot enters the heart, one might feel pain in the chest, arm, neck, jaw, or stomach. The pain can last more than a few minutes, ease, and then come back. Breathlessness, dizziness, feeling sick or breaking out in a cold sweat is common. In the lung, coughing up blood and being breathless are the usual symptoms, but anything out of the ordinary in the chest can occur. In the eye, one loses sight suddenly.

If you think you might have a clot, don't wait around to see if the symptoms change or go away. Call the doctor immediately or go to the emergency room. Blood clots can kill.

To lower the chances of problems, keep active. Move that body! In a pinch, clean the house.

I finally got one perfectly normal blood sugar reading. It was as if my body was working overtime adjusting to the nasty chemicals it was repeatedly assaulted with. By the time I finished the sixth chemo cycle, I would probably be green like the Incredible Hulk. Doubted if I would turn into the bionic woman.

I had my big bottle of Tums; that, along with two pills of generic Prilosec daily, kept my stomach fairly well settled. At least heartburn hadn't burned the corners of my mouth again. Didn't dwell on the fact that my voice was still hoarse and tended to fade if I talked too much.

Did you know shortness of breath can be caused by heartburn or acid reflux? I didn't, but that might have been a cause of my breathing problem. The scenario is that heartburn was catching up to me, but not badly enough to cause shortness of breath except when I was further stressed. That sounded right. When my thighs got stressed, I had trouble breathing. Whatever the cause, my doctor was not terribly concerned that I would turn blue.

At least I did not bruise easily, something that happens during chemo. I'd hate walking around looking like the victim of a beating. Though I could blame Rick—that mild mannered man beating me? Who would believe it without proof? See—here's proof. Nah, no one would believe it, even if I were one big bruise.

Bruising is normally more of an annoyance than anything else but during chemo, they can be more ominous. You can get a honking big bruise (a hematoma) that has to be drained by the doctor. You can get more problems. So model bruises for the doctor. Bat your eyelashes too, if you have them.

Yes, chemo does a number on your blood.

I was measurably more tired in the fourth chemo cycle than in the third. I slept later in the morning—waking up at 10 am rather than 9. Then I would have several good hours to write, clean (don't you dare laugh,) and do whatever. In the third cycle, I would ensconce myself in the living room chair, turn on the TV and fall asleep about 5 pm.

In the fourth cycle, 2 or 3 pm worked better for a nap. I was very tired by then. Depending on how long and satisfying the nap, I either managed to stay awake until bedtime or dozed in the chair. The night I fell asleep four times as Martha and Rick debated new cars I hadn't had a nap and was too stubborn to go to bed at 9 pm.

They talk about chemo causing bone-deep tiredness that is not allayed by sleeping. I could see the point, but my tiredness responded to rest. I just needed lots of extra rest.

The medical community was becoming aware that fatigue is considered more debilitating than nausea by patients. There are medicines for nausea, but not for fatigue. It is described as tiredness, exhaustion, depression, feeling unwell, loss of motivation and limitation of mental state. Over 75% of patients complain of fatigue and in up to a third, it can seriously impact their lives. It can get so bad that the patient doesn't eat well or take care of herself, even forcing delay of therapy.

Be warned; it doesn't magically disappear at the end of ;chemotherapy. It can last for a year or longer. (The fatigue associated with advanced cancer is more complicated.)

One study found that of 218 women with early stage breast cancer, 6% had problems with fatigue after one year. Another study found that breast cancer survivors who ate more omega-3 fats were less likely to have long-lasting fatigue (hooray salmon, mackerel and tuna.)

To fight tiredness, make sure physical causes are treated. Anemia, the pile of pain killers and other pills the doctor prescribes, salt imbalance, and thyroid deficiency are a few of the causes of fatigue that can be medically treated. Inadequate sleep, depression and anxiety also cause fatigue. What cancer patient doesn't deal with those? Once the doctors check the body, turn to your mind to devising ways to improve your condition.

Cancernet.co.uk calls them coping tactics.

- Acceptance: Don't get upset. It's not your fault.
- Eat well: Balance your diet.
  Carbs keep energy up, but skip sugar. Go for whole grain, fruits, vegetables and beans, especially lentils, kidney beans, black beans, peas, garbanzo beans, soy beans, and pinto beans. Lovers of low fat yogurt can gobble away.
- Exercise: Regular exercise is proven to combat fatigue.
  Walking, jogging, dancing, biking, etc. don't make you work so hard that oxygen in the blood is not replaced by faster breathing. The idea is to not have "a negative oxygen balance."
  As the British website says:
  "Other recent studies have suggested that transitory periods of anaerobic exercise are particularly helpful. In practical terms this means pushing the exercise rate briefly to a higher level of oxygen consumption which the lungs can replace at that instance. On stopping, breathlessness continues until the oxygen deficit is restored—this is quite normal and the body is completely used to it. We've all sat on a bus panting for a few minutes after we have had to run for it! Anaerobic exercise has the advantage of opening up the lungs by taking deep breaths, keeping them flexible, compliant and generally in an all-round better condition. It also stimulates the

body's natural erythropoietin hormone (epo) which gives the bone marrow a signal to make more blood. A recent trial, for example, involving women receiving radiotherapy from Michigan showed that those who participated in exercise 20-45 minutes 3-5 times a week had a significantly greater haemoglobin (red blood cells) and lower fatigue that their more sedentary counterparts."
So don't just sit in a chair.

- Distraction: Watch a good movie, listen to stirring music. Go for a drive, visit a friend. In other words, do enjoyable things that will distract you from feeling pooped out. Also, try not to become too hot or too cold. Skip the sauna and making snowmen.
- Rest: Go ahead and nap. If your body needs rest, it needs rest. Try to limit the length of the nap. You don't want to snooze so much during the day that you have trouble sleeping at night.
Do the sensible things that improve sleep. Avoid caffeine in the evening, don't drink huge volumes of anything that make you wake up to use the bathroom. If you are hungry, a small snack might help you sleep. Try to stick to a schedule—go to bed and wake up at the same times, but don't force yourself to lie in bed and wait for sleep that isn't present and accounted for.
One interesting tip that is not always seen is to avoid turning on lights when you do wake up in the middle of the night. Light will disturb the body's circadian rhythm and make it harder to sleep well.
- Task Avoidance: Here is your excuse to avoid running up and down stairs. It won't help. Pace yourself; spread chores out over the day with breaks to rest. Streamline the things you do have to do.

I think the best advice is to do what you can. You are the best judge of your situation. Push through a reasonable amount of work and let the remainder slide. If you had pneumonia, would someone expect you to do this task? Would you expect to be able to do it? Don't be a glutton for punishment.

Whatever you do or don't do, don't bother with guilt. It is a most unproductive emotion. It won't give you more steam and it won't help you face your lack of energy. If your significant other complains of your laziness, shove this book in his/her face and let him/her feel guilty.

Thursday, March 8, 2012

I had others, but since I had given up on the black skull cap, I only wore one winter hat to cover my poor head when I went out. The same hat every time. It was the red knitted winter hat Martha bought me. With the weather getting warmer, this was not going to work, so I started back on the Internet, searching for something to wear. There are companies out there selling hats, scarves and wigs made for the cancer patient although some of them offer very few items.

The American Cancer Society store is www.thehopeshop.org.

www.etsy.com is where people sell handcrafted items. There are crocheted and other hats, hand dyed scarves, turbans, and even surgical scrub caps. I fell in love with an authentic 1920's cloche, but looking at it objectively, I didn't think it would fit. Besides, no one, especially me, said I could spend $500 on a hat.

www.softhats.com has turbans and hats that look comfortable and more stylish than a basic skull cap.

www.hatsforyou.net has a lot of choices.

www.4women.com has pre-tied scarves in attractive materials. They are kind enough to have videos showing how to tie them and one showing how to measure for the correct size.

There are lots of Internet stores—I only listed a very few, and some of those may have disappeared by the time you read this. Do a Google search for chemo hats and see what comes up. If you want to stay more traditional, go retro and get that 1920's cloche or a Prairie bonnet. etsy.com had an authentic Victorian bonnet for $1,600 or so. For summer, a brimmed hat may be a wise choice as chemoed skin may have problems with the sun. Styles to watch for that should cover the whole head include cloches, sun hats, bucket hats, beanies (maybe,) berets (some.)

Or get a scarf. I ordered a semi pre-tied bandana from www.headcovers.com. They have tons of scarves in different dimensions, some kind of pre-tied for fumble fingers, as well as hats, turbans, a few wigs, and cosmetic supplies. False eyelashes for when yours give up the ghost! Fake eyebrows also, as well as templates to help you draw a decent eyebrow.

Or get a wig. There are stores catering to the chemo patient and stores catering to anyone.

The bandana came in the mail promptly and was acceptable to this hater of things on the head, being very light and cool. I might feel funny wearing it in public, so I also got a turban from www.softhats.com. Sadly, it wasn't big enough to fit my fat head.

I admit that at times I was tempted to get it over with and cut eyeholes in a brown paper bag. It is an old, tired joke, but it wasn't an old, tired feeling.

Chemotherapy Cycle 5

Monday, March 12, 2012

It was 2 am; I was being bad. You see, I woke up Friday feeling pretty darn good. My legs didn't hurt, I didn't lose my breath every time I turned around, and my taste buds were halfheartedly working. I had energy! I gloried in health the whole weekend. I felt like a member of the human race and I didn't want it to end, so I was being bad and staying up.

I had to be at Henry Ford Hospital at 9 am to see the oncologist, and then have my 5th chemo treatment at 11. Then I'd be back in the slough of despond—though I was not despondent. It was just the slough.

It was now 4 pm. I was home, sleep deprived from staying up until 4 am and waking up at 7:30 to drag my sorry body to the hospital. But I started Cycle 5.

I gained a few pounds; the guess is it was water weight. My face was rounder. I needed to have the eye doctor stretch the glasses so the stems were not too tight. Again. My head had gone bullet-shaped with tufts of wispy fur, a too narrow forehead and cheeks that bulged like a bulldog. That would get worse, but once I was off the steroids, it should fade away. I had so much to look forward to! I'd like a face that thinned to normal.

My blood work was better than last week. Don't ask why, I didn't and Dr. Medica didn't elaborate. The best part was my immunity didn't drop to the pits. I had not been sick, not even when Martha had the flu. Backtrack a tiny bit—yes, I had been sick, but it was my sinuses, nothing unexpected.

I needed to check in with Dr. Sanatio, miraculous primary care physician, to review the blood sugar thing. My numbers were up and down, not seemingly connected to my diet as much as to my state of health at any point. That was my observation and Dr. Medica pooh poohed it. It had to be connected to my diet; the drugs were out of my system by the end of the first week and thus not affecting blood sugar.

Could I respectfully disagree? If my taste buds stayed wonky, if my fingernails waited until the last week to grow darker, if my legs wobbled all the time, then the drugs were still affecting my system. I truly believed that the ups and downs of my blood sugar were connected in the same way.

That might be stubbornness, but doctors do not know everything. Dr. Medica certainly wasn't in my body. I was. I knew that I ate eight Hershey kisses and my blood sugar went down. Not logical, Mr. Spock, but yummy.

Dr. Medica was concerned about my legs and feet. She didn't want neuropathy to shut down mobility. I promised to get up and move around on a regular basis—keep the blood flowing. Also, I would take B Complex vitamins twice rather than once a day. Give those muscles and nerves as much bolstering as possible.

My toenails were in better shape than my fingernails. Dr. Medica didn't think any toenails were going to fall off. She was noncommittal about the fingernails. They didn't feel loose.

Then Rick and I went to find food. I was predictable; I got a banana, a muffin, and a bottle of apple juice. Half the juice I saved for when we got upstairs. Rick filled a cup with ice and apple juice and I sucked on it when the IV drips started. It did seem to make a difference in the state of my mouth. Not true for everyone, evidently, but for me, the coldness seemed to limit the attack on the mucus membranes of my mouth. (After the fact, I wondered if wrapping fingers around and laying toes on ice packs the first minutes of chemo were a good idea to help with neuropathy. Too much and you would risk frostbite.)

I had a different nurse for every chemo treatment. They were all equally nice. Ask a question and you got a fully informed answer. This time, I clarified flushing.

Flushing is the cleaning out of the chest port with a saline solution. When they drew blood through the port, they manually flushed (washed) it before and after, using big honking hypodermic needles to shoot saline solution through the little lines that had been plugged into the port. Before to make sure it was clean and in working order, since the port had been idle for three weeks between chemo treatments. They flushed it again manually after drawing blood to clear the blood out of the port.

At the beginning of the chemo treatment, I got a bag of saline to puff up my body and flush again. Then I got the Taxotere IV drip. When that was done, there was another bag flush before the Cyclophosphamide drip started. That flush was so the two drugs didn't mix together, which could get nasty. When the Cyclophosphamide drip was done, the nurse manually flushed the chest port clean. Then I was done with the chemo treatment.

Sounds like a lot of saline, doesn't it? Maybe my veins sloshed for a while, but medically it is okay. Some people feel like they are floating when the flush is done. I didn't get that, but I could smell a slightly alcoholic scent from it, which is a hallucination, since it is salty, not alcoholic. The body doesn't understand the process and assigns a smell even though it is wrong.

Once I finished chemo, the port would stay with me. Even if it wasn't used, it should be flushed every month or six weeks.

This time, the nurse set the Cyclophosphamide drip to go faster. This can bother the sinuses, so they usually leave it slower. My sinuses were fine in the fast lane, so the treatment was done a half hour early. Then Rick and I went out to eat.

I visited the restaurant restroom after I ate. Remove the mirror, please. I did not look healthy. My face was pasty and lumpy. Ah well, vanity, thy name is not Ann.

Also, I began drooling from the right side of my mouth. I would not be aware of it, but a drop or so of saliva would wiggle its way out and sit on the corner of my lips. More would follow and the accumulation would go for a walk down my chin. Then I could feel it and wipe it away. This is another facet of mucositis (or neuropathy?). My handbook from the Breast Cancer clinic did not mention it; I found the information on the Internet. So besides looking like a pasty freak, I appeared demented.

Thanks a lot, Cancer.

Wednesday, March 14, 2012

Oh, woe is me. The heartburn was starting.

The bill from Henry Ford said I spent $10,046 in their pharmacy. No, I didn't go on a shopping spree. That was the cost of the chemo drugs they poured into my veins two days ago.

I resented that I had triple negative cancer. If I'd had regular, everyday old tumors, I'd be done with chemo. I could be growing hair, getting my fingernails back into shape, feeling decent. Drinking ice cold, clean tasting water, sleeping normally. It was triple negative's fault that I was still in chemo. But I was absurdly proud that nothing had interrupted the schedule. My immune system hadn't crashed. Neuropathy had not crippled me.

Thursday, March 15, 2012

The heartburn pretty much went away. If I chewed three Tums when I first woke up, my stomach left me alone. Wished I could get the rest of my body to leave me alone as easily. Hindsight is 20/20: don't overdose on heartburn medication. Talk to your doctor and let her find something that works for you.

The darkness in my fingernails shot up right away. Add some on toenails to balance things out. Numbness in fingertips, with sore nails and numbness in toes. My mouth had a metallic taste that cut right through all the beverages I had assembled, so drinking was a bummer again.

I revised my definition of diarrhea. It was not loose stools, it was sludge. It smelled really bad; I wanted to move the toilet to the backyard in the fresh air. Yes, I know that would make it an outhouse. Better an outhouse than stinking up the house as I did. I was a toxic waste dump oozing sludge. (Fast forward to the information on C Diff if this is a big concern to you. Be aware that some of the fatigue I experienced from this point forward may have been caused by C Diff.)

Other than that, I just didn't feel well. I marathon slept. Last night I went to bed at 11 pm. Woke at 8 am and was alive for two hours. At 10 am, I crawled into the chair and turned on the TV. By 11, I was asleep. I dozed off and on for the rest of the day. Woke up when Rick came home about 7 pm. He fed me and by 9 I was dozing in the chair again. Went to bed about 12 pm and woke up at 11 am. Everyone reminded me that the body heals while it is asleep. I felt like Sleeping Beauty, but decidedly not a Disney princess.

Saturday, March 17, 2012

I do believe I felt alive. Yesterday, I was so dopey, I couldn't figure out what to eat. I nibbled here, there and everywhere, not getting a meal until Rick came home and poured food down my throat. With vague hunger pangs in my stomach, I'd stand in the kitchen, staring in refrigerator or pantry, not seeing anything to make a meal. Again and again, I would grab something—cheese or crackers or a piece of bread—and nibble on it. It would barely pacify my stomach, but I was too befuddled to assemble a meal.

I only woke once in the night and got about 11 hours of sleep. I may have felt alive, but I had no ambition. I sat in front of the computer all afternoon playing games. Didn't want to play games, but couldn't think of anything else to do.

Hope I came out of this funk in the next day or so. I had four needlepoint canvases to block and sew into pillows. Sure, they could wait; but then again, they shouldn't wait.

I sent Rick to the grocery store with a few ideas of what to buy to feed my off-my-feed body. All I wanted was sweets. Cheesecake, cookies, pudding, ice cream, candy. I thought I might kill for a Nestles Crunch. I hadn't waved to an Oreo in months. Could I be bad? Yes, but I was afraid to mess up chemo. Protein. I kept reminding myself I was supposed to want protein. It felt like a balancing act between falling apart and becoming healthy. My seesaw was stuck on the wrong side.

The sun was shining, the windows were open and I didn't have a sweater on. It was one of those glorious spring days that Detroit goes gaga for. I sat in the chair and didn't care.

I was still bothered by tics around my eyelids. Wanting more information, I went to the Internet. Ah, it gets so interesting—a reminder that the hip bone is connected to the collarbone. Everything is interconnected and it's hard to sort out what's responsible for what. Maybe a doctor finds it easier.

One cause of twitches is Hypocalcemia, a lack of calcium in the blood. Actually, it is an electrolyte imbalance and if you get it from chemo, it is very serious. If your blood test results indicate you suffer from it, your doctor will closely monitor you.

The symptoms of Hypocalcemia? Nerve and muscle spasms and twitches. Cramps in leg and/or arm muscles. You might have numbness and tingling in fingers and toes. If it gets bad, you can become confused or disoriented. Your heart might beat irregularly. Let it get bad enough and it leeches the calcium out of your bones, bringing on osteoporosis and its headaches.

Best thing to do if you have it? Eat lots of calcium. If the doctor approves, add a calcium supplement to your vitamin mix. Enjoy collard greens and kale, sardines and salmon (with bones,) red beans and seaweed, all rich in calcium. Dairy products are the best source, though. Milk, cheddar cheese and tofu are chockfull of calcium. Many foods are fortified with it.

Other electrolyte imbalances can make you twitch, specifically a lack of potassium, magnesium, or sodium. From advice given on the Internet, your weekly blood test will warn the doctor if you have a problem and action to correct the imbalance can be taken. Electrolyte imbalances are not a bogeyman a person can slay with a magic wand.

Keep in mind that anti-nausea drugs can cause twitches. Stress can do it also. Stress? What stress? Why would a person afflicted with cancer and going through chemotherapy have to worry about stress? (Yes, I could be sarcastic. I earned the right.)

It seemed unlikely that the tics around my eyes, which began slowly and increased over successive treatments, were caused by anything other than chemo drugs. Judging from Internet chat rooms, tics are a common complaint of chemotherapy. Everyone seems to get them around the eyes.

It seems the tics go away after you finish chemo.

Monday, March 19, 2012

Higher energy day. I needed it. Started by going to Cottage Hospital and getting my blood test done. Got home, planning to give Martha the car and sew as much as I could for the day, but as soon as I was home, I had a call from my most illustrious computer client.

Quick explanation is that if they don't print labels, they might as well take the day off—and the monitor for the label computer died. So I made a fast trip to Staples, buying a basic plug and play flat screen monitor (and NO, Mr. Salesman, no matter how much you nag and drag your feet, I do not buy extended warrantees. Clients won't pay for them. I told you, so just shut up and get the monitor.) I got home just as Martha was ready to go to work. Drove her there and went to the client's.

Thank God energy was up and effects on my legs were down. If this had happened a few weeks ago, I would have crawled into the building. As it was, Eddie's smile didn't dim when he saw me; Bill didn't apologize for dragging me out of my sickbed.

Heather was an angel. My hands were not strong enough to pull the monitor out of the box, so she did it. What caused the loss of strength? Not sure, but I hadn't noticed it before. Maybe it was a temporary aberration, but we should guess neuropathy was to blame. I also had trouble with the little screws on the cable connections, but that was more because I was trying to avoid banging sensitive fingernails. Hooked the monitor up and it came on. Ready to go.

Chatted with the boss, Tim, who went through chemo last year. He was in San Francisco last month and had some trouble walking. Neuropathy related. He said it comes on suddenly for no discernible reason; he rests and it goes away. It does interfere with Tim's ice hockey hobby, but I keep telling him that at his great age he should be a referee, not a goalie.

Weakness is not the only residual effect he has. He was pre-diabetic before treatment and the drugs pushed him over the edge. Hoped I didn't end up in that situation, but was pretty sure it was happening to me. Tim commented that I looked good for what I was going through and admired the Gothness of my fingernails. Then the big tease called me Aunt Jemima because of the bandana scarf I had tied on my head. I threatened to go natural and he laughed.

My toes and the balls of my feet were kind of numb. It made driving uncomfortable. I could feel the gas pedal, but didn't want to keep my foot pressed to it. I went home and did a lot of sitting. I was tired, not drop dead tired, but stale. Didn't do any sewing.

That was the end of the pre-tied scarf. Not Tim's fault—he only confirmed my hesitation about the Aunt Jemima look. I switched to the turban I had ordered. It had elastic all the way around, which needed loosening to comfortably fit my fat head, but it looked a little more sophisticated than the bandana. Sophisticated, hah.

The girl next door loaned me a bag of gorgeous silk scarves. I had to return them; they slid right off the back of my head. If I tied one under my chin like a babushka, it would stay put, but I am not my Polish great-grandmother. I discovered I was jealous of all the women on TV and in real life who walk around with scarves or turbans and look pulled together. They have fashion sense. I don't. Please hair, grow back fast.

Heartburn was under control. In the morning, my stomach felt sour, but three Tums on top of Prilosec ate enough acid that I could eat what I liked, even spaghetti with tomato sauce. Eating was enough of a trial; my mouth was not a salt lick as it was last chemo cycle, but there was a steady hint of salt in the back of my mouth, enough to make chocolate taste weird. I watch the cooking shows where chefs rave about mixing sweet and salty, but it didn't suit my palate. If it happened in every dish in the course of a meal, they'd change their minds. Take that, Bobby Flay.

Digressing to cooking shows, I wanted the chefs to cook for me. As Iron Chef America wrestled with mangos, I yearned for them to deal with my reality. The Chairman would plop me in a judge's seat between the grumpy guy and the actress and skip the secret ingredient. Instead, I would tell Cat Cora and the others what appealed—meat with gravy, fried potatoes, nothing that was vegetable, zero enthusiasm for any and all beverages. If they even looked at a hot pepper, I would give them no score whatsoever. Let the Iron Chefs scurry around for an hour creating meals that appealed to the chemoed palate. Wouldn't that be grand? When the show was over, I would take the leftovers home.

I had an intense craving for decent tasting food. It was discouraging. Since December, I had eaten lots of protein, limited sugar, balanced my diet. Drank lots and lots of water and fruit juice so I wouldn't get dehydrated. Turned my nose up at soda pop because there's no nutrition there. My one concession had been chocolate ice cream because it soothed the sore mouth and tasted good. No more. Even ice cream let me down.

Beverages left me unmoved. I could remember water tasting good. Now I would rob a bank to get it; water tasted like it came out of a bog. Hamburger patties with anything didn't satisfy. Goulash was mushy. Ham was salty, corned beef might as well have been unseasoned. Mac and cheese was flavorless. I developed an aversion to vegetables—not just one, but all of them. Fish was absolutely dreadful. Applesauce scared me after heartburn burned the corner of my mouth.

I couldn't care less about nutrition. Protein or carbohydrate—what was the difference? I just wanted something to taste good and nothing obliged.

Sunday, March 25, 2012

Monday went fairly well, but the rest of the week was a slow slide down. Thursday I felt acid in my mouth all day. I made sure I took the Prilosec and chewed more Tums than the label advised. At least I escaped the acid Mt. Vesuvius in my mouth.

My legs started to bother me, but not to the degree they had last cycle. They felt sore, but supported my weight. My hands and feet were a little tingly, a little numb.

My ears were bad. For whatever reason, the sides of my neck felt heavy and tight. I took antibiotic religiously; without it, I would have been sicker than a dog. I also took decongestants at bedtime, something I tried to limit. This week, I had to have them every night. If I didn't take them, I didn't sleep. I made an appointment with Dr. Sanatio for Tuesday. He would help me sort my head out, plus I was supposed to consult him about insulin.

My blood sugar evened out, but the results of each test was a little over normal. I consistently had to give myself the minimum dose of insulin. I was going to be so angry if my body had been pushed into diabetes, but there wasn't any way to be sure until chemo finished. If I could discipline myself to eat a proper diabetic diet—count and limit carbohydrates, no sugar, eat lots of protein, balance each meal—maybe my blood sugar would improve. I just couldn't wrap my head around the diabetic way.

I wasn't drinking enough of anything. As a result, my taste buds deteriorated and I had the metallic taste in my mouth again.

Friday night was a mini-crash. When I went to bed, I sternly told myself, "No decongestant. You don't want the rebound effect to kick in." What is the rebound effect of decongestants? Taking them while you have a cold is okay. Taking them regularly for a longer period of time, one risks having the decongestants cause more congestion. That is the rebound effect.

After years of sinus problems, I learned firsthand about the rebound effect. I had to stop all decongestants for months and was absolutely miserable. Then, I could take them for short periods without rebounding into purgatory.

Here I was, taking them for a week. So Friday night, I didn't take a decongestant. And didn't sleep. Actually, I slept for an hour and then I was awake, sinuses stuffed up, ears ringing. Getting back to sleep wasn't going to happen. I got up for two hours, which is how long it takes to start my sinuses draining, then I went back to bed. And couldn't sleep. After an hour, I got up again and stayed up until 5 am. Then I slept for half an hour.

At 6 am, I took a decongestant and slept until 2 pm. I wheedled Rick into feeding me, watched TV and fell asleep about 6 pm. Woke up at 9, ate again, and at midnight, went to bed. Yes, I took the stupid decongestant, but I didn't sleep all that well.

You decide how much was due to my sinuses and how much was due to the problem of interrupted sleep during chemo. Personally, I think it was as much the fault of the drugs not washing out of my system properly due to my failure to drink enough liquids as it was the fault of my sinuses. They warn you not to get dehydrated during chemo.

What is so bad about dehydration? Your body needs water to function and how much it needs is an exact science.

Normally, you lose 84.5 ounces every day to maintenance of the body, keeping your holy temple at the right temperature, cleansing your innards. Think of it as a daily wash and spin cycle for your organs. Regular food intake puts in 16.9 ounces of water; the remaining 67.6 ounces you need to maintain normal hydration comes from drinking fluids. So minimum, you need 8 eight ounce glasses of water a day for normal function.

Or go by the Mayo Clinic guidelines. They say the 8x8 formula, which is 1.9 liters, is okay because it is easy to remember. More exactly, we need:
- 3 liters a day for men (12½ eight oz. glasses)
- 2.2 liters a day for women (9⅓ eight oz. glasses)

That is for normal function. Chemotherapy ups the requirements. To top it off, you need a waterfall of water to flush the chemo drugs out of your body.

During treatment, you should aim to drink (at a minimum) 10-12 glasses of water a day, not 8. And don't count any drink with caffeine towards the allowance because caffeine leaches extra water out of your body. Forget beer; you shouldn't have alcohol while you are in chemo.

If your immune system is depressed and the quality of water out of your faucet isn't great, go for bottled water. Try different brands because they do differ in taste. If they don't taste good, try a splash of Perrier in your bottled water. Does amazing things.

Side effects get in the way. You lose more water than usual if you have diarrhea or throw up. How about sweating, another common chemo problem? There goes more water. If you have a fever or bleed more, you lose water faster. You are not eating well, so you are probably not getting the usual amount of water from food. You are not drinking as you should, probably because it doesn't taste good—it doesn't go down or stay down well—you are marathon sleeping and not drinking. A sore mouth discourages drinking.

Chemo drugs can remove water from your cells and damage glands that help to keep you hydrated. If you don't drink enough, you have unsafe levels of chemo drugs in your body, which can mess up your liver, kidneys, bones—anything it wants to mess with. Dehydration can upset the electrolyte balances. It might delay your next treatment, which can lower the effectiveness of chemotherapy. You can get Neutropenic Fever—dangerously low white cell counts—which throws you into the emergency room. You can be hospitalized to deal with the effects.

During chemo, a small water shortage produces significant symptoms and consequences. It is a common problem. Here is a list of the symptoms:

- Fatigue/tiredness
- Cotton dry mouth
- Dizziness
- Stiff joints and muscles
- Nausea and vomiting
- Difficulty sleeping
- Reduced mental clarity
- Short attention span
- Difficulty swallowing
- Dark urine or less urine
- Weakness
- Headaches
- Dry skin
- Reduced focus
- Constipation
- Muscle cramps
- Depression
- Irritability
- Reduced energy
- Pain/aches

Sounds like the effects of chemotherapy, not dehydration. My non-medical opinion is that if this list is accurate, the side effects of chemo are worsened by dehydration. If you didn't have the problem before you dried up, you would get it after. And get it worse.

The most dire symptoms of dehydration:

- Severe abdominal cramps, pain or bloating
- Skin so dry it stays in a peak when pinched
- Sudden rapid or irregular heart beat
- Excessive sleepiness with difficulty arousing
- Blue lips
- Dizziness
- Confusion
- Rapid breathing

The good news is that your doctor monitors your weekly blood tests.

Dehydration that creeps up on you should be reflected in the results of your blood tests. The doctor will know about it and take steps to halt the dehydration. If you get bad enough, the doctor's office will call and tell you to make a special trip to the chemo unit for a saline IV.

But if the dehydration process revs up, you might run into trouble before you have your blood test. Then, you could be up a tree. So, if you have problems getting the quota of water into your system, call the doctor. Take their advice. If only to feel as good as possible, do what you have to do.

I was a little dizzy; nothing serious, but that could change, depending on the cause. Dizziness can be a symptom of serious trouble, so I would mention it to the oncologist.

There is an art to dealing with dizziness. As websites advise, I walked slower. If the vertigo got worse, I would have to pick up the throw rug in the hall, keep the house well lit to highlight obstacles, and wear sturdy shoes (ones with less flexible soles.) All are sensible precautions against falling. If I was really unsteady, I would need a walker or a cane to add a solid "third leg."

Carrying a cell phone in case I ran into "Help, I've fallen and I can't get up" was smart. I ran into that problem a couple of years ago when I fell while pruning bushes. I tore ligaments in my left ankle and was totally disinclined to walk anywhere. Scratch that—I couldn't walk. Sitting on the grass felt like a grand idea. The sun was shining, the weather was warm. I could have stayed put until Rick got off work. A neighbor called my husband to come home, which was helpful. She also called the police, which was embarrassing and unnecessary. If I had had my cell phone in my pocket, I could have called Rick myself.

Me, I forced myself to drink extra. Didn't matter if it didn't taste good or if I didn't want it. I made myself drink.

Tuesday, March 27, 2012

Some things never change. Blowing my nose, I got mini nosebleeds. I was tired and my legs didn't feel good. I was out of breath whenever I walked more than five feet. Ears were ringing, toes felt weird, but my fingernails were less sensitive. I tasted a bit of salt with everything and quite frankly, I was not all that interested in food. Not surprising when cheddar cheese potato chips tasted like butter and regular potato chips tasted like vegetable oil.

It's a conundrum why, when the drugs should have been out of my body and my poor abused system should have been busy repairing itself, I tended to feel worse, not better.

I found out that plans were being laid to fly me and Rick to Sacramento at the end of July. I wanted to go earlier! I wanted to go at the beginning of July! I wanted to go now! I had to find out the schedule for radiation before any decisions were made.

A recent development was water retention. I noticed it mainly in my legs—socks left deep indentations above my ankles. The dents would gradually (maybe over a half hour) smooth out.

Went to see Dr. Sanatio, who was comforting regarding blood sugar. He felt it would drop to normal levels once my body rid itself of chemo effects. In the meantime, do my best to watch the carbs, especially potatoes, pasta and bread. He looked up yesterday's blood test results and was quite pleased with their strength.

And yes, when your nose drips, it's in freefall. Thank you, Mr. Cancer, for that attention grabbing side effect.

Thursday, March 29, 2012

Went to the oncologist today. I thought I was doing pretty well, but what do I know? Was I doing well? Yes and no. Overall, I felt dandy, except for not getting enough sleep. But my legs were acting up. In fact, I hauled the cane out of the closet to take with me as a precaution. It was not the shortest walk in the world from the hospital door to the Oncology Department and I thought I might get some use from the cane.

To be fair to Henry Ford Hospital, it is not a long walk for a hospital complex. They thought about all the suckers without hair who were going to have to get there; they put a bank of elevators in a handy spot. It's not their fault I had trouble walking. And yes, the cane was useful. I think I relied on it about five steps out of every twenty.

I was shaky. It just wasn't a good day.

I told the nurse I was shaky and that my legs were misbehaving. My weight was up a good five pounds. Next thing I knew, she was checking my blood sugar. 161. Not the greatest number in the world, but the norm for me right now. So it wasn't high blood sugar giving me fits. No, it was just one of those things that happen when you are in chemo.

Then she checked my temperature and it was about 100°. I felt fine and said so. Believe it or not, by the time Dr. Medica came in the examining room, my temp was back to chemo normal, as in below 98°. Go figure.

My sixth and final chemo treatment was to be Monday. So close and yet so far! This was my last scheduled appointment with Dr. Medica; she added one six weeks down the road.

She wanted me to start taking Gabapentin, an anti-convulsant, for the neuropathy. It is also prescribed for menopausal hot flashes, restless leg syndrome, and epilepsy. I would have to be careful not to take antacids within two hours of taking Gabapentin and my Naproxen had to go in the cupboard because the two drugs don't get along. My legs would stay still at night (they already did) and it could make me sleepy, which was good for a laugh.

The drug was studied (another clinical trial) and found not effective at preventing neuropathy, but it works well controlling the pain of neuropathy. It was being studied as a possible treatment for chemo-induced nausea. Of all the drugs that had been prescribed, Gabapentin was of the least use, in my opinion. Then again, if it made walking a breeze, I would be a fan.

Next, I needed a diuretic because I was retaining water. I loved the name: Hydrochlorothiazide, but not its side effect of weight gain. It causes the kidneys to pass unneeded water and salt into the urine. The list of side effects read like the results of a chemotherapy session.

As a side note, Hydrochlorothiazide masks the use of performance enhancing drugs. Russian cyclist Alexandr Kolobnev was kicked out of the 2011 Tour de France bike race after it was found in his urine. Its greatest sin is it can nudge the body into diabetes. Permanent diabetes.

Third, changes to the Metoprolol (blood pressure medicine) prescription. Take it twice a day instead of once a day because it wasn't handling my blood pressure well and my heart rate was increasing. Not soaring, but increasing. Buy a blood pressure monitor that also registers heart rate. Use it and email the results to Dr. Medica for three days.

I should have kept my mouth shut. My blood pressure was not dangerously high—153 over something—and that could have been caused by the stress of walking on wavering thigh muscles. But I also told the doctor about the times I lay down to go to sleep and my heart beat fast for several minutes. Ah well, better safe than sorry.

But the blood pressure monitor cost $60 and I was trying to hang on to money, preparing to help Martha move into a condo at the end of April. I'd rather have had money in the bank than a blood pressure monitor that would probably only be useful for a week. Hindsight is 20/20: I still have that stupid monitor and still need to use it once in a while.

I had more tests in my future: a chest x-ray, an echocardiogram, a mammogram and ultrasound of the left breast only, a fasting blood test for sugar and cholesterol. I also had a new doctor, a radiation oncologist, to make friends with.

Sometime soon, I would start radiation therapy. We didn't get into that in any detail; Dr. Medica preferred that the radiation oncologist discuss it with me.

Dr. Medica did another physical exam of my left breast. I reminded her that I had felt something there before the last visit. She had felt it also, but then it disappeared on her. She found it; it's probably a cyst. It better be a cyst.

We didn't spend a lot of time talking. I didn't get a lot of explanations, but it was a busy day.

The last thing that happened was another nurse showed up with an oxygen meter. It's the little clip they stick on your finger that measures how much oxygen is getting to the tip of your finger. This one also measured my heart rate. The highest oxygen number you can get is 100; I was at 97. The nurse complimented me on that number. Then, we went for a walk around the floor, just so I could get out of breath for the nurse and the doctor who happened to be in the hall. He was watching the way I walked. Uh, huh.

When my legs bothered me, I tended to walk looser, as if I was on a boat, rolling a little. Lock the knees and let the calves flop. It made walking easier but it probably did look a little weird. I hoped the doctor comprehended this.

The results of our walk were interesting. My oxygen rate did not fluctuate, but my heart rate went up as I got shorter of breath. When we were done, I went to the pharmacy to spend $60 on a blood pressure monitor and then home.

And on the Internet. If you search Google for "heart rate goes up as you get short of breath," the first entry is about COPD, the breathing disorder. But if you stick "Chemotherapy" in front of the phrase, you learn about Dyspnea, a condition where you experience shortness of breath. For heaven's sake, why the silly Latin name? No matter, Dyspnea can be caused by heart problems, which I didn't have, lung problems, which I didn't have, or anemia, which I could have, courtesy of chemo.

So maybe Dyspnea was making it hard to breathe when I walked. Not sure, but anyone could develop it.

chemocare.com listed the symptoms:

- Overly tired
- Fever, chills, or headache

- Pain in muscles or lungs
- Being awaked in the night by shortness of breath
- Coughing spells

- Wheezing
- Tight chest, difficulty getting a good breath
- Trouble lying flat
- Bloating/water retention, especially in feet/ankles
- Chronic cough

What do you do about Dyspnea? Try to exercise to keep your body as fit as possible. Even ambling around the house is better than doing nothing. Don't smoke or drink alcohol and avoid pollution and common causes of allergies, like mold, dust mites, and pollen. Raising the head of your bed six inches with bricks or using 2-3 pillows might make it easier to sleep. Use relaxation techniques to keep anxiety at bay.

There are bunches of types of Anemia. We are worried about a low red blood cell count in the blood. The symptoms:

- Fatigue
- Increased heart rate
- Disturbed vision
- Shortness of breath
- Lightheadedness changing position quickly
- Headaches
- Dizziness
- Weakness
- Chest pain
- Pale skin

Anemia is common in poorer countries, especially among menstruating women. What do you do about it? Do what those poor women can't: eat plenty of protein and vitamin-rich foods and drink those fluids. Until it improves, avoid activities that make you short of breath or make your heart pound. Plan so you can achieve as much as possible without keeling over. Rest between activities. Ask for help getting things done.

If the anemia is serious enough, the doctor may give you another prescription or have you take iron supplements. (If it's a liquid supplement, the taste is gawd-awful.) Above all, finish your chemotherapy and be patient while your body builds up your blood. Anemia is not a life sentence, but restoring normal blood levels is a slow process.

Friday, March 30, 2012

Got a series of phone calls from Henry Ford Health System setting up appointments.
- Mammogram and ultrasound of the left breast on April 11
- Meet the radiation oncologist April 12
- Echocardiogram April 18

They were all at Cottage Hospital, close to home.

I went to Cottage and had my blood test done. Then I toddled over to the Women's Center and set up an appointment for the bone density test that Dr. Medica said I should have done. They scheduled it for the same day as the mammogram.

On the way home, I stopped to buy a Mega Millions lottery ticket. The jackpot was at a record breaking $640,000,000, the largest jackpot in history. Sure would be nice to win. We could buy a condo in Sacramento, buy loads of antiques, do all sorts of things like go to the Titanic exhibit.

The Henry Ford (formerly called The Henry Ford Museum and Greenfield Village) had the traveling exhibit about the Titanic. I heard about it last year and marked it on my calendar. It was the exhibit that the Ghosthunters show investigated—evidently it is haunted. Wanted to go, definitely wanted to go. Not now; I'd never make it into the building. Hoped I felt better before it left in September. It didn't seem likely.

Sunday, April 1, 2012

Woke up feeling okay, but not well. Guess I didn't get an energized day before the next chemo treatment, which was tomorrow.

No, I didn't win the lottery.

I had sewing to do and discovered that my fingers didn't work quite as well as they should. I couldn't grasp the thread and pull when I was picking out a seam. I had to cut the thread with scissors. It seemed like a combination of strength and sensation got in the way. My fingers couldn't hold the thread tightly and I couldn't feel where the thread was on my skin. That is neuropathy, folks, minus the disabling pain many people have.

Katie pulled an April Fool's joke on me, the skunk. Every year, she gets me. The first year she was in Sacramento, I was scheduled to fly out there on April 2nd. She called me April 1st, asking why I didn't get off the plane. I went into a panic, thinking I had mistaken the day of my flight.

Tonight, Martha brought her laptop to show me Katie's first tattoo, a line or three of Lord of the Rings elvish writing on her arm. I went ballistic, as both girls knew I would. How many times had I told them, "Nothing permanent. No tattoos, no piercings." It was henna, not permanent at all. Katie got me good.

I wasn't even aware it was April 1st.

We were having trouble with the insurance about the bill for the PET scan. They said it was investigational in the treatment of my breast cancer and not covered under our insurance. I had it done for the clinical trial, I guess. Was it a four way, "Who is going to pay for this?" The hospital, the clinical trial, insurance, or us?

I was slightly constipated. Bet it was the diuretic. I lost five pounds in the last two days, thanks to it. But once the water was off, I didn't want to take the pill. I could monitor my weight and if it jumped, I'd take one or two—enough to control the water retention but skip the constipation. Overall, I preferred loose as a goose over tight as a gander. (Behaved and didn't stop the pills.)

I was supposed to gradually up the dosage of Gabapentin, the anti-convulsant for the neuropathy, to a total of three pills a day. I noticed a distinct improvement in my feet, hands, and legs while taking one pill a day. I had to talk to the oncologist and ask if I could stay at that dosage.

Can you tell I dislike taking a ton of pills? Gabapentin only deals with pain; it doesn't do anything to heal neuropathy. If one pill managed the discomfort to my satisfaction, why take three?

Chemotherapy Cycle 6

Monday, April 2, 2012

I started Cycle 6.

Last cycle, last chemo treatment. Where's the confetti? And turn on the Hallelujah Chorus and the 1812 Overture!

I woke up with my legs working well; I had a feeling today would have been the day of energy and normality. Instead, I was going to Henry Ford Hospital's Chemotherapy Unit.

I was wearing one of my trusty chemo shirts and a pair of cords, loose socks so I didn't get dents on my legs (like it or not, I still needed the water pills,) and ratty tennis shoes. No bra. The bra straps sat right over the chest port and would only make hooking me up a pain. It was cold enough to wear a winter coat and the red winter hat that looked best on my pear shaped head.

While Rick and I sat in the hospital waiting room, he fielded several calls from work. Thank God this was the last time he would have to take time off to babysit me; he was really needed in the office. Bless Joe, his supervisor, who firmly agreed that taking care of me was more important than the company. Joe's wife, who I mentioned before is an oncology nurse for Henry Ford, probably filled him in on the importance of support.

The nurse weighed me and was pleased I had dropped eight pounds. Water pills are wonderful. They should be issued to brides three days before the wedding, given to females the day before Homecoming and the prom, and to all mothers attending special events for their children. It is great losing those last few pounds that make the outfit not quite fit. Thanks to treatment, I couldn't have cared less how my clothes fit.

The nurse, Pam, took me straight to the chemo room. My blood test was done on Friday, so we could skip it. Rick headed downstairs to the coffee shop to get apple juice while the nurse plugged the IV into my chest port and started the anti-nausea drip.

He was back and had apple juice ice ready for me to suck before the Taxotere drip began.

Pam set up a follow-up appointment with Dr. Medica. It would be May 9th, two days after our wedding anniversary. My, how time flies. When Rick and I married, I never thought about 30 years—I didn't think ahead at all. I sure didn't think I would celebrate my 30th wedding anniversary chemoed, scars all over my left side, and no hair. Please, could I feel good that day?

The nurse was confused; was I to come in the next day for a Neulasta shot or not? I had never had one because my immunity didn't skydive, so we guessed not.

I asked for a copy of my blood test results. I had not gotten them every time, but it was helpful to keep an eye on my figures. She printed it out and I stuck it in my bag. It was better to go over it at home, in front of the computer, so I could look everything up. Who can remember what each thing is? I sure couldn't.

Remembering the PET scan bill, Rick asked to speak to Trish, the clinical trials lady, if she was available. She was; she would be in soon. Rick read, I played a card game on my Kindle, and Taxotere dripped into my vein.

Trish showed up within the hour. No, the PET scan was not done just for the clinical trial; the insurance should have paid it. Could I scan and email the letter from the insurance to her and she would look into it? Yes, I certainly could. Somebody had to save us from this expensive bill. (Many moons later, I found out that Henry Ford Health System wrote the bill off. We never had to pay it. Thank you.)

Then it was time for the Cyclophosphamide drip. That was the drug that attacked my mouth. I sucked apple juice ice for nearly ten minutes straight, determined to spare the sad mucus membranes in my mouth as much as possible. The roof of my mouth had felt shiny and slick for the last two cycles; now the sides of my mouth and the gums had begun to feel the same. Mucositis was going to be a big problem with this last cycle. God forbid I got sores in my mouth.

I went back to my Kindle card game. Playing cards is good for killing time. It helped to block the sounds of the Chemotherapy room. I hated those sounds.

The buzzer went off. Chemo was done. Pam came, unhooked me, and reminded me that when I came in for my follow-up appointment with Dr. Medica, I should have my chest port flushed. Then she gave me a card to celebrate my completion of chemotherapy signed by all the nurses. I got a hug and I cried a little. (I cried again when I wrote this. Lord, I hate chemotherapy.)

Rick and I hightailed it out of the chemo room. I did not look back.

We went to our favorite bar for burgers. I recalled hearing about a woman who went out to eat after every chemo session; I now knew that wasn't special. If she could go out to eat one week after every chemo session and actually enjoy her meal, I would be impressed. I'd find her and beg for the secret to her success.

No big success here. I wasn't spared. By nighttime, my voice was going. My taste buds were fading. I had no appetite at dinner. When I took my pills, the water didn't taste good.

The side effects were kicking in early.

Tuesday, April 3, 2012

I hate it when I'm right. Side effects were jumping my bones. Woke up feeling dull. Took my pills and the water tasted muddy. Lazed in bed for a while, then decided I should get up. I had no appetite; I ate some bottled peaches only because I knew I should have something. Tested my blood sugar. It was up to almost 200, nowhere near as high as I thought it would be.

Feeling blah, I did all the things I did to manage chemo side effects. I was so blah, I couldn't bother to eat.

By midafternoon, I knew I needed fuel, preferably a meal. Any fool knows a few peach slices will not do for a whole day—I was being foolish. Browsing in the cupboard, I pulled out a package of Pasta Roni Parmesano. It was not good nutrition, but the last time I had some, it tasted okay. Cooking it and cleaning up the kitchen a little, I realized my sense of time was off. The noodles were boiling long before I thought they should be. Then the kitchen was decent and the noodles were ready to eat.

They had no taste at all. Grape juice had no taste. This was pure and simple chemo hell.

I sat in front of the computer. With no energy, what else was I to do? I played Pogo, wished I felt well, and then remembered to look over my blood test results.

Go figure. My white blood cell count at 13.6 was higher than average. Chemo is supposed to depress it.

The RDW (red cell distribution width) count was way high, which meant nothing to me. Trying to understand this, I found a web site that talked about RDW counts. Evidently, if you compare the RDW count to the MCV count (MCV is mean corpuscle value) how they relate together gives you something to bite into. A high RDW count with a matching high MCV count means a folate deficiency. My soaring RDW count was matched by a low MCV. Ahh, normal MCV combined with high RDW can signify a B12 deficiency. It seems I might have a vitamin B12 problem, though I was taking my Super B Complex faithfully.

Neutrophils usually go down when you take chemo drugs. This is a cause of reduced immunity. Why would mine go up? Higher neutrophils are a sign of acute inflammation (a chemo bugaboo) and sometimes a sign of nervousness.

The number can be raised by drugs such as Cortisol or Prednisone (neither of which I had taken.) Wait, Cortisol, a steroid hormone, is released by the body naturally in response to stress and a low concentration of glucocorticoids in the blood. Not that I understood all this, but it can increase blood sugar. Is that where my need for insulin came from? From sensitivity to this natural steroid?

The only other information that I could find that made any sense was that a higher neutrophils count is a response to a bacterial infection. This was beyond me. Let Dr. Medica analyze it.

My monocyte count was high. The first web site I found said that monocytes are a part of the white blood cells, thus dealing with immunity. A low count is good, an elevated count means a problem. If it were really high, it would probably mean I had Leukocytosis.

What is Leukocytosis? It's just a fancy name for elevated white cell counts in the blood. Wikipedia kindly tells us, "Although it may indicate illness, leukocytosis is considered a laboratory finding instead of a separate disease," and, "It is very common in acutely ill patients." I can buy that. The most common cause of leukocytosis is a bacterial or virus infection or parasites. Cancer can also cause it, as can a whole host of other problems such as anemia, asthma, kidney failure, heart disease, severe stress, and poisoning. (I voted for poisoning.) Again, I would leave this for Dr. Medica to worry about.

My serum albumin was a little low, but that seemed to indicate that I hadn't been eating enough protein. Also, the BUN was under average; if it was high, it could be a problem.

My cholesterol levels stank. I found a mention on the Internet that chemo drugs can throw them off. Once I got done with all this, I'd ask for another test.

Despite delving into the Internet, I failed to get a total picture of my status from the numbers. The lesson to be learned here was that blood test results are too complicated for the layman to decipher. Ask the doctor if you are concerned about yours. I trusted Dr. Medica; let her worry about red flags.

T-shirts spotted on the Internet

- I pay my oncologist big bucks for this hairstyle
- Chemo is my drug of choice
- You can't scare me—I've been through Chemo
- Go ahead, poke my port
- Chemo ate my eyebrows
- Not only is my short term memory horrible,
  so is my short term memory
- I have Chemo Brain. What's your excuse?

There were others, but I didn't think them clever. If I habitually bought t-shirts, I'd get "Go ahead, poke my port." It's snippy, kind of how I felt.

Thursday, April 5, 2012

Lousy day, callooh callay. My mouth was a mess and I had the energy of a pea. I was back to the salt lick; everything tasted overly salted, even when I wasn't eating.

Amidst the misery, I got an email with pictures of my great-great-grandparents attached. They are now the only photos I have of that side of the family other than one of my great-grandfather. Angeline looks sweet and John Wesley has the long straggly beard that made men of the mid to late 1800's look like hermits. His picture verified that my mother's and brother's blue eyes came from that family. Shape of the eyelids is the same and as far as you can tell from a sepia (that brownish yellow color) print the blue is the same intensity. Thank you to the Swartout family for sharing invaluable pieces of my history.

Life goes on, however. A bathroom pipe sprung a leak; we had plumbers in, wrecking our savings account. One of the plumbers knocked the ceramic towel bar off the wall and dropped something in the pedestal sink. We glued the towel bar back together and complained to the boss. They brought a new pedestal sink and installed it. It was about the cheapest you can buy—loads cheaper than the broken one. It doesn't suit the style of the bathroom or house and the pedestal was ugly. Worse, the guy drilled a series of holes in the ceramic tile wall to get it in. If I hadn't been so chemo dopey, I wouldn't have let him do it.

I was so out of it, I didn't look at what the guy was doing until I heard the drill making holes in the tile wall. I looked, was aghast at what I saw, and figured it was too late to complain. Never using that plumber again. Hopefully never doing Chemo again either.

Monday, April 9, 2012

Don't be fooled by the last post or two. I was truly amazed how different the sixth cycle was from the other five. While the side effects kicked in early, I did not feel as sickly, I had more energy, my mouth did not get coated with the white paste that wouldn't brush away. True, I lost my taste buds, but only the tip of the tongue got sore.

Still, don't let me fool you. It wasn't a picnic. Yesterday was Easter. Rick and Martha went to church. I didn't even consider it. Easter dinner? Never thought about it. Colored eggs and candy? You have got to be kidding.

It was difficult to banish the metallic taste—usually I would drink a ton of water and the medicine taste would go away. This time, nothing banished it. Between the salt lick and the drug slick, even chocolate tasted lousy.

I craved foods: cheesecake! We bought one and it was okay. Not spectacular. It vaguely tasted like cheesecake with strawberries on it but it could lose the strawberries. Oreos! I ate a few. Hard to chew, being fresh, and they hurt my tongue. Spinach dip! Can you believe spinach having no taste? I gave up and fantasized about being able to eat anything I wanted and having it taste the way it should.

There was grit on my teeth. After each chemo treatment, before mucositis took control of my mouth, a gritty film coated my teeth. Brushing banished it, but it would return within an hour or two. Scraping my teeth brought up a pasty substance that reminded me of plaque—or what I imagined plaque to be, since I had never seen that dental no no in such quantity. If I didn't keep this white junk cleaned off, it hardened within a day or two along the gum line. It coated my bottom front teeth the most. I used a dental pick to carefully remove it, although I did not always do a very good job of scraping it off. Occasionally, I would pick hardened bits of grit out of my mouth; it was as unyielding as stone. (Yes, it was plaque.)

Besides that, it was difficult to clear bits of food out of my mouth. Think about the process. When you eat, bits of food get stuck various places, don't they? That is why you have toothpicks, fingernails, and business cards. Eat a chicken leg, dig shreds out from between molars with a toothpick. Pull that spinach strand through your front teeth with your fingernails. A gummed up bit of bread stuck along the curves of your molars? Pop it out with a stray business card. That is how the healthy (uncouth and impolite) person tends to dental health between brushing sessions. Don't count on it while you are in chemo.

Your mouth is such a mess, you don't notice food stuck in your teeth. Even if you are fairly certain you have a half inch chunk of chicken leg crammed into the space between your molars, you can't feel it. Why? Your tongue is sore and slightly dead. The food locating radar is turned down or off by mucositis—plus running a sore tongue along teeth is self-inflicted torture. It feels like you are stropping your tongue with a saw-toothed steak knife.

The answer, of course, is frequent application of toothbrushes, toothpicks, dental picks, dental brushes (like miniature bottle brushes. If you don't see them in the store, ask your dentist,) and water pics that can crawl between the teeth and clear crud away. Easy does it—your gums might bleed from a poke that normally does nothing. There is no sense irritating your mouth more than it already is and you don't need to risk infection.

Reevaluate the brand of toothpaste by your sink; some sting like the devil on a raw tongue, if nowhere else. The experts recommend a mild toothpaste with fluoride, not mint.

The same advice goes for commercial mouthwash. Use your noggin before you are too miserable to go to the store. Most mouthwashes contain alcohol and should not be used during chemo. Find a mouthwash that is alcohol free and milder. Water it down or don't use it at all. Replace it with baking soda (one quarter teaspoon) and salt (one eighth teaspoon) in a cup of warm water. Store it in a covered plastic tub by your toothbrush for up to a week. Pretend to be James Bond with his martini—shake to mix—and swish as often as you wish. It actually soothes the sore mouth. If anyone has the gall to complain that your mouth doesn't smell minty fresh, you have my permission to breathe hard in their face.

Do your best to keep your mouth clean. It will help avoid developing sores and infections and make your mouth taste as good as possible when nothing tastes good. If your mouth gets bad enough, the doctor might delay your chemo treatments to allow it to heal. Delayed chemo means less effective chemo.

This cycle, there was no indigestion, heartburn, or uneasy stomach, and the diarrhea was not as nasty. My rear could tolerate regular toilet paper, though I had a package of Cottonelle wipes still to use. It would outlast the diarrhea, I was sure, guaranteeing comfort in the nether region. I do believe that my biggest success in treatment was in the avoidance of hemorrhoids. Aren't you proud of me?

I had less trouble sleeping at night and needed fewer hours napping. I still got short of breath and tired, but not nearly as much. It wasn't debilitating. My skin peeled; my forehead was a mess. The palms of my hands turned vaguely white; I had dried up and blown away. My fingers and feet were perhaps a little more into neuropathy, but not much. I stubbed my big toe and could ignore the pain in my toe but my toenail felt like I had dropped an anvil on it. My Goth fingernails had not gotten measurably worse.

My blood sugar seemed to be stabilizing—I got a reading of 104 (excellent) one morning. I had hopes of throwing away the rest of the blood pressure medicine. I considered not purchasing a new bottle of Super B Complex vitamins when I finished what stood on my bedside table. (Don't do that! Keep using B vitamins indefinitely. Bolster those nerve endings any way you can.) I didn't need Prilosec or Tums. I had enough Refresh eye drops to keep my eyes flushed until I reached a drug free state. I had antibiotic to stabilize my sinuses and ears.

This cycle was easier on me. Did they give me a lower dose of drugs? No.

I believed it was my imagination made my body powerful. It squelched the effects of the drugs. It wriggled endorphins into all the seams of my desperate self that were hurting from the poison and made every atom feel better. If my body didn't do it, my mind did. Maybe. I didn't know the cause. I was merely grateful for relief.

I inspected my hair. The top of my head was depressing. Remember, Martha cut my hair an inch long before it all fell out. (Misstatement!!! It did not all fall out. Just most of it—enough to justify saying it all fell out.) What hair was left was now white. Not a pretty white, but flour white. There were dark hairs scattered all over my head, but they did not show from a distance. My head looked a bit like someone had dusted flour over it and my scalp, which was totally visible, was pasty white except for a reddish vee along the top where the sun had permanently darkened the skin along my accustomed part.

Martha claimed she could see where my hairline belonged, but a thorough analysis said she was delusional. I could feel stubble where hair had broken off at the scalp. It was accompanied by this strange white hair that hadn't grown much beyond the original one inch length. Using the magnified side of the hand mirror, I could see there were hairs growing in the wrong places, namely on my forehead, not within my hairline.

Have you taken a good look at Donald Trump's hair on a bad day? How it looks crinkled? Mine looked worse. I could not imagine this hair growing out dark, curly, or luxuriantly, not to mention silvery. This was a low blow to my vanity; to understand it, let's take a trip down memory lane.

I was born with dark hair. It darkened as I grew older. My brothers had thick, black, curly hair—mine was diluted to nearly black, straight, and fine. I looked like a redhead in strong sunlight, thanks to the highlights in my almost black hair. After Martha was born, the miracle of hormones made my hair thicker, and if not precisely curly, there was a nice wave in it.

I began graying in my twenties; the gray was mostly in front at the temples. I boasted that it looked distinguished, as a man's silvered temples are considered distinctive. In my thirties, someone commented, (and I never forgot,) "When you go completely gray, your hair is going to be that lovely silver color." That person was correct. Thanks to lavender shampoo, which discouraged yellowing, my gray hair was silvery white.

As silver multiplied, I lost red highlights, until I was left with a plain almost black background for my mane of silver.

Menopause stripped the thickness and most of the curly wave off my head. My hair was closer to my original almost black, fine, hair, and the gray went a pretty white with silver highlights. It was acceptable, attractive enough that I seldom considered dying it. Did it once, liked it, but never did it again.

Then came chemo. "Hi O, Silver, away!"as the Lone Ranger said. After six sessions with lifesaving poison, my hair looked like Donald Trump's with flour white replacing silver white. Life is not fair.

As you can see from my flight of vanity, I had started thinking about the rest of my life. Chemo would soon be a bad memory and I could get on with my life. It would be nice if I had a presentable head.

The only benefit I received from chemotherapy (other than killing cancer so I could stay alive,) was that somehow or other, I lost almost forty pounds. Through the ups and downs of water retention, appetite loss, and all the other stresses, I shrank my stomach and managed to lose all that weight. Clothes I had put in the bottom of the drawer and the back of the closet because they were tight were now loose. My chemo shirts were laughably big. My daughters urged a new wardrobe, but I would wait to see if I managed to keep the weight off.

I began researching radiation therapy. That would begin soon enough and I wanted to be prepared. Knowledgeable.

Thursday, April 12, 2012

I have taste buds! Food tastes like food. Water tastes like water. Kind of. Oh, happy day. You see, Mr. Loathsome Cancer, you don't have your teeth in me. I am well on the way to health. My determination to be rid of you is not diminished and I can see the end of the effort down the road. I look forward to a cancer-free life.

I went for a bone density test. Last time it was done, I had fat bones. Hoped that remained true. (It did.) Then I had a mammogram. Ouch. It hurt more than it used to. Bet the inside of my breast was still trying to settle down from the lumpectomy. I had heard of women who failed to get timely mammograms because of the pain. Mine hurt and I still did not understand that mindset. A few moments of pinching is infinitely preferable to chemo.

The radiologist came in to talk. She wanted to verify that two sites had been melon balled out. The mammograms (a hefty number of pictures) were completely clear. The only thing worth mentioning was what she called a post-operative area. I had to assume that this spot was clearly post-operative since she saw no need for an ultrasound of the breast. Dr. Medica would get a report. If she was unhappy about not having an ultrasound done, she would holler. I assumed. I hoped. I trusted.

Mammograms had become a touchy subject. I was unhappy that they only did the lumpectomied breast, not both. I would schedule one for both breasts on October 1st. Vigilance!

I had difficulty walking, though I did well enough getting around Cottage Hospital. Leaving the Woman's Center, I stopped at the drug store. I grabbed a bottle of Aquafina out of the cooler, then went all the way across that huge store to the aisle that held the Olay products. By the time I got there, my legs were shaking and I had trouble breathing. I found the box I wanted and then decided I had to get out of the store before I fell down.

I made it to a chair outside the pharmacy section, sat, and waited for my breath to even out. Darn, I needed one more item. Rest, go get it, then head for the checkout, which was blessedly free, pay, and get to the car. I sat for five minutes, resting my aching legs and restoring my breathing, before starting the engine.

Once in a while, I had trouble maintaining balance. This seemed to happen most often when I was walking and turned my head to the side. My body wanted to follow my head, but was going in a different direction. I always managed to catch myself, but I gave Martha and Rick a few nervous moments. If it continued, I would check with the doctor. (It went away.)

I had to go to the basement for backing material for a needlepoint piece. I got down the stairs okay, had the material in hand quickly, and then struggled up the stairs. I was afraid I was going to have to go up on my butt, but made it on wobbly legs. I plopped into the chair in front of the computer and stayed there for quite a while.

I had trouble pulling my driver's license out of the case. I couldn't grasp the plastic with my fingertips, and that was the only way to get it out. Giving the cat a pill, I had trouble hanging onto that tiny white tablet. Martha asked me to feel a spot on her arm. I had to decline because

I wouldn't have been able to locate the bump. It was all the fault of my fingertips, which were somewhat numb. Not completely numb; I could hold a large needle and sew, I could button buttons, but I lacked fine control and the finer feelings. To get silly, my fingers were as insensitive as a man with no romance in his soul.

This neuropathy disability was not extreme. I was in no danger of scalding fingers unawares. My legs functioned enough to escape a burning building. Sometimes my legs worked perfectly well; my fingers responded to orders. They were not painful, nor were they uncomfortably numb or tingling when at rest. They didn't keep me up at night. They didn't cause me to pop painkillers. I didn't require physical therapy. I was luckier with neuropathy than I ever have been with lottery tickets.

The neuropathy might fade away, as the nerves affected by chemo regenerated.

Nerves have remarkable powers, filling in (pot)holes, fixing frayed edges, growing what they need to function. If they are upset by a salt imbalance or some other cause, they can be calmed. It's a matter of patience while they heal, a slow process, somewhat akin to a committee finding a solution. Eventually, I might be back to normal, perhaps in a matter of 3-5 months—if not longer. Please note the word "might." Dream away, but it doesn't always happen. Sometimes neuropathy is a life sentence.

Chemotherapy-induced Peripheral Neuropathy is one of the most common side effects of chemo. It is also one of the most common reasons for abandoning treatment. The nerves affected usually deal with touch, heat or pain. I obviously had the touch kind the most.

There are clinical trials being conducted to address it, so hopefully it will become a thing of the past. For now, if your neuropathy is severe or painful, there are options.

Ibuprofen reduces chemical signals along the irritated nerve that cause pain and inflammation, so if you need something for minor pain, it would be a good choice over aspirin or Tylenol. Other medications ease symptoms and banish pain. Physical therapy can do wonders to restore movement.

Don't suffer in silence. Keep detailed records of your difficulties and take the log to your doctor. He isn't going to doubt that you have neuropathy and he has a host of treatments to suggest. Join support groups, learn about solutions to problems. Include diabetes in your searches—lots of diabetics suffer from neuropathy. Watch out for quack solutions. This seems to be an area where the nuts go wild. And may the force be with you.

I still needed a daily nap. Health is not automatic, nor is it quickly gained once lost. Still, I was pleased. There were no interruptions to my chemotherapy treatment. It was never postponed; all went on schedule. That offers the best chance for a cure.

If your treatment isn't seamless, remember the phrase, "Mind over matter." It works for others, why not for you? Scientists at CalTech and UCLA had individuals manipulate the behavior of an image on a computer screen by thought alone. True, the research study was more involved than just asking people to think about changing a picture, but they had a 70% success rate. The test subjects succeeded in using their minds to control a computer screen.

Sound impossible? Switch to sports figures. They frequently use their minds to improve their performance. Lots of sportsmen talk about visualizing the goal. Arthur Ashe's moment was in the 1975 Wimbledon Final against the favorite, Jimmy Connors, when he stunned the crowd at breaks by pulling his towel over his head and meditating for 60 seconds. Clearly refreshed and inspired, he played the game of his life and won.

Hypochondriacs make themselves sick. Medical placebos work when they should do nothing.

Mind over matter might work. Make this your mantra:

I am stronger than you are, Cancer. You are going to lose this one. Concede your loss.

Tell me you didn't believe this! Myths about cancer

- The type of bra you wear or the tightness of other clothing increases breast cancer risk.
- Exposing a tumor to air during surgery causes cancer to spread.
- Needle biopsies can disturb cancer cells and cause them to spread to other parts of the body.
- There's a miracle cancer cure…

Radiation Therapy

Suggested Shopping List

- Aloe Vera—pure, no additives or fragrances (check the label)
- Clothing that touches the breast may get stained—plan accordingly

Wednesday, April 18, 2012

Dear Cancer,
I am two thirds done with the treatment to get rid of you. Are you shrunk? Better, are you dead? I sure hope so. I'm going to make sure of that with radiation.

I am happy to report that chemotherapy did not do me in. My stomach is still sensitive—I guess the tendency to heartburn will plague me for a while and neuropathy will be a lingering irritation, but you did not beat me to a pulp. I will regain my energy eventually.

Here's spitting in your eye, Cancer. Someday, the researchers will figure out a better way to defeat you. There have been some promising finds. Until you are a thing of the past, we will claw you out with tiger's toenails if necessary.

Just don't assume I was up to par. Martha bought her own birthday cake; Rick and I sang the birthday song and helped her eat it. It was too sweet. I had a present I purchased online stashed in the bedroom. It wasn't wrapped, but at least I remembered it was there. Rick dragged it out and Martha opened the shipping box in lieu of tearing off colorful paper. It was a most uninspiring birthday for an awe-inspiring daughter.

Yesterday, I met with the radiation oncologist at Cottage Hospital. My appointment was for 8:30; imagine my surprise when I was the only patient there. Everyone knew my name. Everyone was uber nice.

I imagined that some research study showed that smooth, congenial interactions with medical staff offers higher survival rates among cancer patients and Henry Ford took it to heart. That may sound cynical, but how else can one explain never seeing a frowning, impatient nurse? Henry

Ford Health System, I commend you. Research or not, all those pleasant people do help one through torture. All those smiles made me feel lighter, less like a sickly freak.

I had to fill out a form that included emergency phone numbers. Thanks to the wonder of speed dial, I couldn't recall Rick's cell phone number. It popped into my head later, so I told it to the nurse on the way out.

After that ignominious start, I was ushered to an examining room and spent several (did I say several? I grossly underestimated) minutes with one of the nurses, of whom there were two. They called themselves partners. Sometime over the next thirty visits, I would even learn their names.

Nurse One went through my medical history. You know, the drugs I took, what surgeries I'd had. They had my miscarriage as an abortion. They missed when I had my jaw broken and reset; that was before Katie was a twinkle in my eye.

Then Nurse One handed me the medication list. Wow, it was fifteen times as long as it used to be, or so it seemed. The steroid called Dexamethasone was thankfully in the past. And I had cut out the Omeprazole, which perhaps was a mistake, but enough of it. (Ended back on it later.) She had me taking an estrogen blocker and I told her no, I wasn't.

It bothered me when, at the end, she ran through the list of my "conditions." No, I was not diabetic—that was caused by chemo. No, I didn't have hypertension—same thing. No, I didn't have acid reflux; I had chemo-induced heartburn. No, I most certainly did not have COPD (which Dr. Medica never mentioned to begin with.) That was breathing problems connected to neuropathy. I got tired of blaming chemo for the ailments currently afflicting my body. Were these diagnoses listed in my records as ongoing problems? Would I have to explain them to every doctor I saw for the rest of my life? Grrr.

I'd admit to mild curvature of the spine, recurrent sinus infections, and almost gone glaucoma, but nothing else. The scary thought was that they didn't expect these problems to disappear once I finished treatment.

Nurse One had me put on a robe. She inspected the skin around my left breast. I told her I was still fighting a yeast infection. I used the powder Dr. Medica prescribed until I thought it was gone, then it would reappear. She told me to stop using the powder—if they felt something needed to be prescribed, they would prescribe it—and gave me directions for the care of radiated skin.

Taking care of the skin they are shooting extra strong x-rays into is the highest priority when you have radiation treatment (hereinafter called plain old radiation.)

The skin gets unhappy. It thinks it is sunburned; it burns to a crisp (exaggeration, I hoped.) Every day, three or four times a day, I should slather the whole area with pure Aloe Vera (you can buy Aloe Vera with additives, so watch for pure,) but don't use it the morning of treatment. Every night, before bed, apply Aquaphor to the nipple area and the various scars (one from the lumpectomy, two scars from surgical tape, and one scar kind of in the armpit where they removed two lymph nodes.) She gave me a baggie with written instructions and several small tubes of Aquaphor.

Aquaphor is a petrolatum based (AKA Petroleum Jelly) ointment made by Eucerin, a division of Beiersdorf AG. It is available in two forms, Original and Healing Ointment. Both versions are similar to Vaseline, but contain extra ingredients. The Original Ointment contains mineral oil, ceresin, and lanolin alcohol. The Healing Ointment contains mineral oil, ceresin, lanolin alcohol, panthenol, glycerin, and bisabolol. Like Vaseline, it is an effective treatment for minor cuts, scrapes, burns and dry and cracked skin. It can stain clothing but who cares if a nightgown or two got ugly? Stain everything! A new wardrobe would be reward for finishing this endless treatment.

I had a vague memory of the doctors instructing my mother to use Eucerin on her skin. Aquaphor appears to be my generation's answer to the ravages of radiation.

If I needed more Aquaphor, there was a coupon for it in the baggie. Oh, and please do not use any other kind of lotion. No deodorant. No perfumes, no nothing. Use warm water, gentle soap like Dove or Ivory, and pat dry. Don't scrub the skin. And don't shave under the arms. A razor could cut the skin and healing could be a problem. If you absolutely must, use an electric razor. Wear a soft loose bra, if you wish, but no underwire bras. Watch out for harsh laundry soap. Lie down and lift the breast to dry and air out the skin often. No letting sun shine on it (there go my plans for nude sunbathing on the Cote d'Azur.) A low cut shirt might expose some of the upper breast, so be modest. Forget that you own a heating pad or a cold pack. Treated skin is more sensitive. You don't need burns or frostbite.

I had to sign my soul away on some forms. Nurse One joked that I had just given her $1,000 because I didn't read the forms. I told her that if she could find $1,000 to take, she was welcome to it. I recognized consent forms and had no need to read them.

The radiation oncologist came in: Dr. Solaris. A man with a great sense of humor, we discussed treatment in general. I would have thirty days of radiation spread over weekdays with weekends off. The side effects

I could expect were skin problems and fatigue. Fatigue because the body kicks into overdrive to heal the damage radiation causes.

My radiation would not touch the heart, but it would skim a portion of the lung. It would not be enough to give me problems, but it would be visible on x-rays as a spot. That was something to remember for the future, if I ever had lung x-rays.

He agreed I would be clear to go to California anytime in July. Enjoy the vacation.

There still wasn't anyone else there. I had the full attention of the Radiology Unit at Cottage Hospital. How nice. And planned. Yes, my being the only patient there was planned. They needed to do a lot to get me ready for treatment.

Nurse One turned me over to Nurse Two; she took me and my too small hospital gown to play with the CAT scan. This first meeting with the machine was a "simulation." Yep, that's what the experts call it—a simulation. The CAT scan would plot the radiation beams for my treatment. The radiation oncologist would use the measurements gained to plan where the radiation would hit and how long it would soak in.

I had to remove my left arm from the gown and lie on the table with my arm raised on a curved ledge. Since I had no problem with mobility, Nurse Two pushed the ledge to a higher position, pulling my arm higher. The oncologist placed wires covered with tape around the breast tissue, which extends farther than the casual observer would believe up toward the chin and over into the armpit. The tape was yellow, like police caution tape, but the edges were cut into triangles. I supposed that, if nothing else, they counted triangles to locate specific sites on my breast.

Dr. Solaris asked me to turn my head to the right and lift my chin as high as possible. The reason for this was that the radiation would be delivered from the right side coming down; he didn't want it to cut through my chin. This was the only uncomfortable part; my neck muscles were stiff and didn't like holding this pose.

Once I was taped up, it was time to run me through the CAT scanner. It's a donut a foot or so wide, and plenty big enough that there was no sensation of claustrophobia. It wasn't noisy either. The table slid me back and forth, back and forth, until the scanner had all the data needed. It didn't take long. When it was done, I was still not to move. Nurse Two had to tattoo me. X marks the spot. Or rather, dot marks the spot.

Tattoos. I spent years ordering my daughters, "Nothing permanent. You can't do anything you can't get rid of," like piercings or tattoos. Here I was, breaking my own rules and getting tattoos. Three of them, to be precise. One on each side of my breasts and one on the breastbone. One tiny dot in each place for them to use to line me up with the radiology machine.

It used to be that tattoo ink was not as permanent as it is today; Nurse One told me they used to ask people not to wash them for weeks, to make sure they didn't fade to nothing. And while inking the tattoos into my skin on the sides was not painful, the one over the breastbone hurt because it was close to the bone. She had gone so far as to visit a tattoo parlor to see if she could improve on technique, but there is no better way to mark the skin.

All these kids who get tattoos are suckers for punishment. I got three tiny pricks, they get trillions. It must burn like the devil.

I could begin radiation the following Monday. I had my pick of appointments and chose 10 am as being late enough to be awake and at Cottage Hospital every day. The way I had been sleeping, an earlier time might be hard to manage five days a week.

I was there all morning. I went to Janet's for lunch. Not because I had a burning desire to go out to eat. Rather, our power was out, thanks to very high winds Monday. I heard on the radio that Detroit had the distinction of being the windiest place in America with the wind steady at 55 mph. Of course our power went out. We ate dinner at a restaurant, read by kerosene lamp, and went to bed with flashlights. Rick woke up to the alarm on his cell phone and he woke me for my appointment.

The power came on an hour after I got home from lunch. Thank goodness, I had a freezer full of food. It was safe. It did not melt. I threw out the milk, eggs, and mayo, etc., figuring nothing else would kill us by growing bacteria. I regretted the sloppy Joe meat; I wanted to eat that. Then I took a nap. I woke up about 4 pm, read my email, read a book, and fell asleep somewhere around 6:30 pm. I crawled out of a bad dream about 10 pm and Rick fed me dinner. Wow, two naps in one day.

I went to bed and slept five hours. Fatigue from radiation would pile on the residual fatigue from chemotherapy.

Thursday, April 19, 2012

I went to the dentist. Perhaps it was too soon after chemo, but I couldn't stand my garbage mouth any longer. The toothbrush just couldn't get my teeth clean. So I made an appointment, telling them they couldn't dig in my gums, but they could achieve something.

They did. The hygienist was careful around the gums, but she picked a ton of plaque off my teeth. Evidently the gritty film I struggled against was indeed plaque; they could not come up with any other explanation for it. They assumed chemo made my mouth dry and the dryness produced plaque. I said that if anything I had an excess of saliva and they shrugged. It's one of life's little mysteries.

The dentist checked my mouth. He said I was lucky; chemotherapy often damages the bone and the root of teeth and he saw no sign of problems. He could see mucositis on my tongue and on the roof of my mouth; please let it fade quickly.

My teeth felt smooth, that wonderful after-the-dentist smooth. Clean. My mouth still tasted bad.

Friday, April 20, 2012

I was sick of the thought of chemotherapy. Radiation was the coming thing; it deserved attention. I didn't realize it was so complicated—I thought gathering data about radiation would be like discussing lumpectomies. It wasn't. It's more like chemo side effects. Endless. Want an information dump? Here you go. It's a hodgepodge of information for a complicated subject.

The purpose of radiation is to eliminate a tumor or to relieve symptoms from a tumor that can't be removed. When can't it be removed? If a tumor is pressing on the spine, or growing in a bone, it hurts, but can't be removed. What if it is in the brain, causing headaches—paralysis—seizures? A tumor near the esophagus can interfere with eating. Radiation can shrink the tumor and ease the pain, the seizures, or open the throat so someone can swallow.

About half of all cancer patients receive some kind of radiation therapy. It can be done before, during, or after surgery and there are three ways it can be delivered into the body.

- External beam radiation is when a machine shoots radiation from the outside into the body in the form of high power x-rays or gamma rays, but not kryptonite. Different doses are needed to kill different types of cancer. This is the most common treatment for breast cancer and the method chosen to treat me.
- With Internal radiation the doctors insert radioactive material into the body at the site of the tumor. It doesn't require surgery; the material can be injected with a needle or slid through a tube, depending on where it is going. The material might remain in the body forever (the radioactivity goes away) or it may have to be removed.

- Systemic radiation involves inserting a radioactive substance into the bloodstream or having the patient swallow it. The miracles of science have found ways to guide the substance to where the tumor cells are and zap them but not others.

If all the choices about radiation come in threes, no wonder it is a complicated subject.

Which of the three methods of radiation is to be used on your body is up to the doctors. How do they choose? It depends on a bunch of factors like the type and size of the cancer, it's location in the body, and how close the cancer is to healthy tissue that is sensitive to radiation.

How far into the body the radiation needs to travel makes a difference—if it is near the skin, external radiation won't have to dig a deep path to the tumor. If it is in the middle of the body, that laser beam of energy might do too much damage to the overlying body parts while getting to the tumor.

The intended victim's general health and full medical history are considered, as well as whether the patient will have other types of treatment, like chemo. The radiation oncologist takes all this into consideration when he decides how to zap you.

And no, it won't make you radioactive. No transforming into mutant Ninja Turtles. It's nothing like the atomic bomb (you won't explode over Hiroshima) or the power plant powering your light bulbs. There is no risk of becoming a walking Chernobyl.

The only people who should skip radiation are pregnant ladies and perhaps those with Lupus. Pregnant women because the doctors can't guarantee radiation spray won't harm the baby. (Get out the hose and wash the car. Listen to your neighbor scream because you watered inside his house when you sprayed the hood and roof. Radiation sprays like water.) Lupus? Past studies indicated that radiation was dangerous for Lupus sufferers, but thought is changing on that. If you have Lupus, get educated—educate your doctors, if you must—figure it out. Sorry I can't give a better response, but the authorities seem divided on Lupus, from what I saw.

If you have concerns about radiation, you should discuss your case with the doctors. Do it well before treatment starts so if changes need to be made, they do not conflict with other choices. Think of treatment like a jigsaw puzzle. Change one piece and the whole board alters.

For example, if you prefer internal radiation—say the radiation center is 200 miles from your home and daily visits would be nearly impossible—it had best be decided before you have surgery. I have a niggling feeling that doctors are not very flexible in the decision; they know more about cancer than the patient and it would take earthshaking concerns to change their chosen path to health.

Plans can be made to minimize difficulties, even with an endless stream of daily appointments. Ask for help, not just from your medical team, but from neighbors and relatives, the American Cancer Society, churches, your local Kiwanis or Rotary club, the local newspaper, an altruistic local business—from anyone you can think of.

Whatever is getting in the way, get creative with it. There is a reason why everyone knows the expression, "Where there's a will, there's a way." It's because we can find a way. If you can't find it, someone else will.

Sunday, April 22, 2012

Tomorrow would be my first radiation treatment. Not really knowing what to expect, I continued researching.

Radiation kills cancer cells by messing up the cell's DNA so the cell can't reproduce and grow or by creating charged particles called free radicals that do the same thing. Radiation may also directly kill the cells. The broken-down cell remains are eliminated by the body and voila, no cancer!

Like chemo, radiation also kills good cells, so careful plotting is needed. How much radiation any particular body part can take is known, so if they have to hit the lung while going after a breast tumor (as in my case,) radiation oncologists know how much the lung can stand without significant damage and plan accordingly. Killing a lung to save a breast is counterproductive, but slightly damaging the lung and saving the patient's life is acceptable.

Sometimes the treatment includes thermal therapy—heating the cells to perhaps make them more sensitive to radiation. That is not widely available; it is being studied.

Normally, after a lumpectomy, the whole breast is radiated. Gee, that is what would happen to me. After mastectomy, radiation is recommended if the tumor was large, or if it invaded lymph channels, the blood vessels, or the skin. If the removed tissue didn't have a nice clear margin, radiation might be indicated. It all depends on if your doctor thinks you are at higher risk of cancer recurrence. Triple negative breast cancer and its propensity for coming back to bite must put it high up on the list.

But they won't do both breasts if cancer was only found in one. Radiation doesn't keep cancer from starting. It kills cancer that is already present.

The only thing I had to do to prepare for radiation was to make sure my skin was clean. No deodorant, no perfumes, no lotions, no ointments. They can leave a film on the skin that can interfere with the rays. No no no!

Monday, April 23, 2012

I drove myself to Cottage Hospital for radiation. As instructed, I used the valet parking service; it is at most twenty feet from the Radiation department. Walk in, go to the right, and open one of the pretty wooden double doors and you are there. The reception area is nicely laid out. It looks more like a lawyer's office than a hospital. The receptionist remembered me and said to go right in and get changed.

Back into a hospital gown, though I didn't have to take off my pants. I didn't even have to remove my shoes. I changed and sat in the waiting area, but it didn't take more than a minute before one of my nurses came to get me. Hah! Nurse One was Mary, Two was Eileen. They aren't nurses, but radiation therapists.

They showed me where they would be while the radiation machine shot me. Across the hall from the bathroom, it was a long narrow room with a counter, several computers, and a monitor focused on a sheet-covered examining table with a slightly inclined top half. If I had any problems during treatment, I should wiggle the fingers of my left hand—or open my mouth and holler—and they would stop the machine and come in to me.

Then they took me to the room across from the changing room. The Room. The door was about 4 inches thick, but I didn't have to try to open it. Go in, swing around to the left, and I was in a pretty good sized room with an examining table in the middle for me to recline on. It was the table I saw in the monitor, of course. I could have asked for a bunch of grapes to munch and pretended to be a decadent Roman, except for the honking huge machine lurking behind the table.

I took my left arm out of the gown; just like the sun, the radiation machine works best on bare skin. I lay on the table with my head in the head cup and my bottom on the seam between the flat and reclined halves of the table. A wedge under my knees eased my back and kept me from sliding down the table. My left arm was up in the holder, my feet were banded together, and my head was to the side. The whole idea was to keep me in the exact correct position.

Mary used a pen (not a Bic and not a roller ball. It is a special paint pen with rather pretty lighter blue ink that is the devil to wash off) to mark where the tattoos were. Then they used the sheet under me to drag me around, lining up my tattoos with red laser lights. The laser on my right side was coming from a panel like a flat screen TV against the wall. I assumed the other tattoos lined up with similar panels to the left and above, but I wasn't supposed to turn my head to look for them. I looked later. Yep, another flat screen on the left. Above me, on the ceiling, a plus sign was cut out of the ceiling tile. I couldn't see the laser through that, but it was there.

Tug, roll my butt a tad to the right. They obviously had lots of practice lining folks up.

The therapists were comfortable talking to me while they pushed me around; they chattily told me what to expect from the machine. The huge arm with a bigger round flat screen would be at my right side, shoot me (painlessly!!! I absolutely promise, it is painless) and then swing over me to the left side and do the same thing.

Okay, I was in position. Eileen covered my right side and stomach with a towel. My left breast was bare. It was important that I did not move. Do not move.

Eileen and Mary left for their control booth. They talked to me through a speaker; remember, don't move. The treatment was going to begin. The arm of the machine moved.

A different arm came out from the middle of the big arm and taking position to my right, took a picture. No flash and I didn't have to smile. The picture was of my innards; they would take one once a week, to check that my breastbone and all other pertinent parts hadn't sunk into my spine or inflated like the bratty kid in Charlie and the Chocolate Factory who blew up. It's a check to make sure the machine is lined up properly with the body. Then the camera arm retracted and the big arm got ready.

I had this large round screen up close and personal with my right side. I was leery of watching it in action, but it won't hurt your eyes. Behind the smoky glass was a set of grills. They looked somewhat like the grills in the wall that the air conditioning/forced air heating system uses except the slots in these grills were flat and gray.

Each time the machine whirred, the strips of the grill moved. Then I could see that they were actually individual teeth that slid up and down, not a stationary grill. The teeth formed patterns going across the grid. As the treatment proceeded, the teeth slid up and down, changing the pattern. Obviously, the patterns corresponded to different parts of my breast receiving differing amounts of radiation. The grills moved down a little, and then the machine whirred for a minute. After the whirring stopped, the grills moved up and the machine whined. Then it buzzed.

I got four whirs on the right side, and then the machine went over my head to the other side and repeated the process. When that was done, all in the matter of a few minutes, one of the therapists came on the speaker and said the treatment was done. They came in, helped me off the table, and set it up for the next victim. I got dressed.

I met with Dr. Solaris again. This would be a weekly meeting of minds. There wasn't much to deal with; it was too early in the process for there to be any concerns. Then I got to leave. Henry Ford Health System politely paid for the valet parking.

Radiation would be given in daily doses over a period of thirty days, with weekends off. Why not one huge dose all at once? First, that would be hell for the skin and hard on everything else (like my lung) to tolerate. Second, just like chemo, they wanted to spread out the treatment to catch a multitude of cells at different stages of growth. Don't kill an adult and leave the baby to grow. Catch the cells at each "year" of growth—maybe a preschooler is more susceptible to radiation. Or a sweet sixteener will collapse and die quicker. Or a cell will "give birth" to more cells just before the third treatment. Let's get those suckers.

Because you are trying to catch the cancer cells at different stages of development, you don't want gaps in treatment. Getting to the radiation center five days a week for six or seven weeks may not be the easiest thing to do, but try not to skip days. When one treatment is promptly followed by the next, the damage to the cancer cells is steady (think relentless) and you're more likely to kill those cells. Don't waste the effort. Take your hangover to the table; it won't do you in. They won't mind if you have a cold. If you have to miss a day, it can be added to the end of your treatment, but the more days you miss, the poorer the outcome.

The medical staff will do everything possible to keep you going, especially if your skin objects to radiation, but extreme problems are rare.

Eileen told me about one woman who started radiation and then started talking to her pastor. They prayed and the woman decided she was healed. She stopped treatment and died of cancer shortly thereafter.

I reminded myself not to lose sight of the goal. Radiation was another of those hurdles to the goal of being healthy. Hopefully, it was the last hurdle, with cancer-free health being the end result. (Safely out of chemo, I was back to my track and field analogy. It fit so well with how I felt.)

When I got home, I slumped in front of the computer for a while. That radiation session was not physically difficult, but my brain wore me out. Finally, I remembered I was supposed to put Aloe Vera on my breast. My word, the skin at the tip of my breast was a little pink. Aloe Vera fixed that right away.

Tuesday, April 24, 2012

The second radiation treatment was exactly like the first, except I noticed more details. Up on the wall was a computer monitor with my name in big letters and a bunch of numbers. The numbers told Eileen and Mary how to set up the machine for me.

At the head of the table, the head cup, a basic padded circle covered with black leather, had different slots it could be positioned in. They put the head cup in the slot that matched my number. The same for the arm holder, only it had a sliding gauge that put it at the right place for my arm and could be placed on the right or left side of the table. Pretty nifty, huh?

Mary told me they used to make a Styrofoam mattress for each patient. The mattress would line them up for the machine, but it was tedious to make and prone to breakage. Flaking? Can't you see a patient going home every day with bits of Styrofoam stuck to them? The thought of reclining on it made me cringe. Imagine listening to Styrofoam creak. The only thing that would mask that would be fingernails going down a chalkboard. This table was a huge improvement over a Styrofoam mattress, even one covered by a sheet.

Wouldn't it be great if a 3-D printer could make a custom designed bed for each patient? It's the 21st century—should take advantage of it. Then again, 3-D printing is expensive. I'd rather spend the money finding a cure for cancer.

Down to business. I noticed more details. The table rose at least three feet. I got four whirs per side, but the whirs didn't match. They were not all the same length and the sound varied. So I asked.

No, they were not the same. Some of the zaps were for closer-to-the-surface breast tissue; those were not as high intensity. Other zaps dug down deep in my breast, so they were stronger. Also, the tip of the breast tends to get more radiation than everything else and they do things to compensate. If one could see the rays, it would be easier to imagine, but they are not visible.

When I got home and smeared Aloe Vera on, I examined my breast. My nipple was definitely affected; it felt harder and looked upset. There were streaks of swelling—yes, streaks. In a two inch radius (a circle) around the nipple, the skin looked pitted and was pink. Aloe Vera soon got everything looking and feeling better, but just wait. Daily radiation was going to make my skin unhappy. What would be the side effects other than that?

Which site of the body is receiving radiation tends to determine what kind of side effects are experienced. Since the scope of this book is breast cancer, I will stick with that subject. Not everyone suffers side effects, but if you get them, treating them quickly is key.

What are the side effects of breast cancer radiation?
- Armpit discomfort: mostly because it is close to the area being radiated and the skin rubs
- Chest pain: the nerves get swollen and irritated
- Fatigue: the body is working to heal. All that energy has to come from somewhere
- Heart or lung problems: The body is stressed, so the heart or lungs can be stressed
- Lowered white cell count: and the associated lowered immunity

Shorter than the chemo list, isn't it?

Remember my mom's experience with radiation. They burned a hole through her chest that never healed. Her heart was nicked, bringing on mitral valve failure decades later. Technology has changed, as you can imagine.

Today's computerized machines are more accurate than those used in the 1960's, allowing the radiation oncologist to aim effectively. They can miss the heart, but it is common for a tiny bit of lung to be radiated. That little bit of damaged lung should not be enough to produce symptoms; it is the overall effect of radiation on your system that can bother the lungs and become a side effect.

With external radiation therapy, the skin is the most affected, at least in the patient's point of view. It will turn pink, red or tan. Women with large breasts (like me) tend to have more trouble; try to keep the area under the breast dry. The skin will get dry and itchy, maybe moist and sore in the folds. Try to avoid skin against skin both under the breast and around the armpit. Plan to baby the skin and expect pain. Well, hopefully not pain, but discomfort. You don't escape discomfort with radiation.

The breast may swell from fluid retention; a larger bra may be called for. If you see indents from the bra, you definitely need a larger one. Sleeping on your back helps the fluid drain at night, but it is back the next day. Tenderness of the breast may crop up—it won't last forever, but massaging the breast lightly may help. Watch out for the skin if you massage. The rubbing might cause a problem.

You won't lose what hair you have on your head, though underarm hair may disappear. You won't get nauseated unless you work yourself up to a state of anxiety that causes it. You should be able to work because the fatigue is not disabling. After chemo, radiation is a breeze.

There are changes in the breast that go on for a year, if not two years, after radiation is done. Skin redness gets out of town quicker than a gunslinger avoiding the sheriff, but swelling of the breast acts like it wants to have a shoot-ut at the OK corral. Though the skin may look normal and the breast starts to feel normal, you can still see changes in a mammogram for up to two years.

Radiation during or right after chemo does produce stronger side effects. It makes sense; chemo weakens the body and radiation weakens the body. Start out weak and the progression is accelerated. It does not last forever, though. Keep good thoughts in mind. It can't last forever.

Recovery from radiation comes in stages. There should be immediate relief after ending treatment, but then it slows down. Some people have residual discomfort, ranging from a twinge once in a while to outright pain. It comes from irritation of the nerves, swelling and scar tissue, rubbing, and sometimes from infection. Physical therapy, gentle massage, medication, and meditation can help. Don't be shy about asking for help.

The ribs can become more delicate from radiation. They can break more easily. I remember my mother sneezing and breaking a rib. Don't forget that was in the 1960's. It is much rarer now. But the treated breast may not gain weight equally with the untreated breast, so if you get fat, you might not be balanced. Then again, you may be the only one to ever notice a difference. No one's breasts are perfectly the same anyway.

Side effects down the road (sometimes years down the road) include a new tumor. Yes, radiation can cause cancer. It doesn't happen often; it can probably be called a rare event, but there is a risk. Radiation to the whole body (versus just your breast) is when it is really harmful.

Tumor, schumor. The risk of radiation is squashed by its value. Since doctors can't guarantee that surgery removed the cancer completely, or that chemotherapy killed all the cancer cells, radiation is another opportunity to remove little bitty tumors from your body. Research has shown that those who get radiation tend to live longer, and live longer cancer-free, than those who don't put up with it.

Sometimes cancer grows again. A person who had radiation and then goes through chemotherapy with a recurrence of cancer can experience what is referred to as Radiation Recall. The breast that received radiation may develop a bad sunburn. This has happened up to fifteen years after the original treatment. Stay out of the sun, don't do tanning beds, and ask the doctor what you can do to relieve pain.

Once you have had radiation on a site, you probably cannot repeat the process. The healthy cells have had all they can take. Of course, if breast cancer hit my right breast, it could have the full regimen, since only my left breast was treated.

On breastcancer.org, Marisa Weiss MD, says, "Cancer cell growth is unwieldy and uncontrolled—these cells just don't have their act together like normal cells do. When normal cells are damaged by radiation, they are like a big city with a fire and police department and trained emergency squads to come and 'put out the fire.' Damaged cancer cells are more like a disorganized mob with a bucket."

Because your immune system can take a beating from radiation, keep to a good diet. Avoid deli foods, thin skinned fruit and all the stuff that was a no no during chemo. You aren't healthy yet. But food tastes better now, doesn't it?

Thursday, April 26, 2012

Fourth radiation treatment. Nothing changed except I realized they had a nurse available—Karen. She was right there near the main door. I showed her my black fingernails; they were lifting more. A couple of my toenails were at risk for lifting themselves right off my toes. She said the lifting might continue for a while. Yes, some of the nails could still come off. Cutting them short might help. Yucko.

What do you wear during radiation? Not a tight bra, that's for sure. I am not sure if a bra is a good idea at all. Check with your radiology team for their recommendation. I reminded myself that I grew up with the group that burned bras and went free. Out in public, I tended to wear my chemotherapy shirts. They were loose, highly patterned, and didn't advertise my freedom.

When the skin under my breasts got sweaty, I tucked old handkerchiefs between my breast and chest wall. They tended to fall out, but did help with sweat. If one were determined (or desperate,) a length of soft unbleached muslin could be tied around the middle under the breasts. A soft t-shirt could be worn and periodically tucked under the breast for a moment. The idea was to keep sweat off the skin.

Friday, April 27, 2012

I woke up feeling better, but tired quickly. Tomorrow would be a doozy; Martha was moving into the condo. I would miss my curly head moppet, though she'd only be 15 minutes away.

There were so many things I could think to do to help, but I couldn't do most of them. Radiation might be easier than chemo, but I wasn't healthy yet.

This would be the last daily report on radiation. It was my 5th treatment and progress of skin damage was so slow, it would be boring to both reader and me to go through each day.

Rick helped me smear Aloe Vera and Aquaphor on at night. I asked Eileen how far he should go with the goop and, using the machine to locate the edges of the treatment area, she lightly marked me with her paint pen so Rick could see where to glop me up. She said how nice it was that he would help. I was surprised. Why wouldn't he?

She told me about a man who had radiation on his back. He couldn't reach to put anything on his skin and his family refused to help. He was reduced to smearing Aloe Vera on a wooden spoon and scrubbing at his back with it like a back scratcher. Eileen told him to bring the tube with him; she or Mary slathered him up every day after the radiation machine was done.

If your care providers are as helpful as those at Henry Ford Health System, you can overcome oodles of difficulties.

Yes, my skin was reddening. No, Aloe Vera no longer cleared it up completely. Though I tried to let it dry before I put on my nightgown, when I woke up in the morning, the material would be glued to my skin. Weird sensation.

Thursday, May 3, 2012

We had a storm last night. Evidently it took out the power to the radiation machine at Cottage Hospital. When I arrived for treatment, they asked me if I could wait a few extra minutes; the technician had it fixed, but had to go through a testing procedure. Of course I could wait. It wasn't all that long a delay either. I only read a few articles in the newspaper.

Nurse Karen was off that day; Jennifer sat at the nursing station. I asked another question. Was it the fault of the radiation that I was ever so slightly nauseated all the time? It had been going on for days. No, the radiation shouldn't have anything to do with my stomach. Still, I had very low level nausea. Jennifer would check with the doctor.

I couldn't get away from side effects. Now I had what felt like a vaginal yeast infection. I picked up Monistat at the pharmacy and prayed for quick relief. Nothing in this world is quite as unpleasant as a yeast infection, at least to this girl. I picked up more Super B Complex and Centrum Silver vitamins, Aloe Vera, and Cottonelle wipes, and ordered more Omeprazole. The pharmacy was doing well by me.

One day of radiation cost $1,680.00. One day!

Wonderful weather. It was so warm we opened up the porch, which means French doors in the living room opened wide on a screened porch. Almost like being outside. I love it. No matter what house I lived in for the rest of my life, I wanted French doors I could leave open. Forget sliding glass doors; they just don't have the same effect. Please note that I noticed the weather. A month before, it would have gone over my head.

Monday, May 7, 2012

Happy Anniversary, Rick! It was our 30th wedding anniversary.

I was alive to enjoy it, though my thoughts didn't go that way. I didn't get the feeling that I had dodged death. I had been sick, but not deathly ill. At least that was how I felt in May, 2012. Death by cancer was not—nor had it ever been—on the agenda. (Forget what I wrote in the beginning of this book, please.) I had been dealing with a nasty condition in the best way possible, which wasn't very pleasant, but sometimes you have to do things you don't want to do, right?

Now I had been married 30 years. Wow. What would the next 30 years be like? Better than the last six months, please.

Thirty more years would put me in my mid-eighties. I would outlive my mother and grandmother, but not Grandma's cousin. Lalie died at 105. I could live long enough to have a 60th wedding anniversary, as could Rick. It was unimaginable, just as 30 years of marriage was unimaginable when we got married.

We celebrated with a steak dinner; a serious celebration would be later. After all, I didn't feel well. Why didn't I feel well? Well, beyond the slightly upset stomach, Saturday I had diarrhea all day. Enough that I lost four pounds, gained a new hemorrhoid, and was miserable. Finally, I took Imodium to stop the diarrhea and got constipated.

Today, I got a little dizzy when I went into the Radiation Center. Karen, the receptionist, gave me some orange juice, which took care of that. But then I told them about the diarrhea. So I got to see another doctor, Dr. Solaris not being in.

I have large breasts; rarely, in large breasted women, the blood can be affected by radiation to the breast. That could cause nausea. Again, it is a rare happenstance. The doctor advised me to take the nausea medication that was prescribed for chemo and see how I did.

In addition, they ordered a stool test, the diarrhea equivalent of a urine test. I wasn't sure what they wanted to check. Thanks to chemo, there are a number of things that could be wrong. I was given a round plastic tub the size of a Cool Whip container, with arms connected that allow it to fit over (or under) the toilet seat. I was to defecate into the container (no urine please,) screw the lid closed, and take it in to the lab. Don't refrigerate!

In the meantime, I was still a little nauseous.

Friday, May 11, 2012

Wednesday I had my six-week checkup with Dr. Medica. I was weighed and remembered to remind the nurse that my chest port needed flushing. She said they would do that at the end of the appointment, in case blood tests were ordered.

I had to change into another of those trendsetting hospital gowns, this time with the opening in back. Then I saw the trainee doctor. He went over the list of my medications, dull topic that it was. And Dr. Medica came in.

She checked my toenails and pronounced them fine. She inquired as to the state of my diabetes, and I told her the sugar blood tests were slowly falling into normal range. We ran through the other major complications I had earned from chemotherapy and she pronounced herself satisfied that I was doing well, though she didn't believe me when I told her that the neuropathy was not painful. Dr. Medica mumbled something to the effect that my attitude was suppressing the painful nature of the condition.

She examined my breasts and lymph nodes, looking for lumps. As to the diarrhea, she thought I might have suffered a bout of food poisoning. The test would tell.

The most serious part of the appointment was her discussion of a study that was done some ten years before. The surprising result of the study was that following a low fat diet lowered recurrences of triple negative breast cancer by about 50%. She wanted me to concentrate on a low fat diet and on losing weight. I would certainly try.

As she told me before, I needed to be most vigilant for the next two years. After that, I still needed to be vigilant for the following three years. (I'd be vigilant the rest of my life, thank you.) For now, I would see her every four months.

Every day I felt a little better.

C Diff

Thursday, I went for radiation. Pulling up to valet parking, I saw radiation therapist Mary talking to the valets. I went in and was surprised to see everyone, as in Mary and Eileen, congregated in the lobby, talking to the receptionist. They greeted me and we went into the lab corridor, only to find the lady doctor and the nurse clogging the hall. I wasn't to change for treatment, but was to talk to the doctor first. Uh, oh, what had I done?

It wasn't what I had done, but what my treacherous body had done. Call Terminex ASAP! I had bugs!

Bugs in my intestines, as in bacterial bugs. Thanks to chemo, antibiotics and radiation, or maybe antibiotics, chemo and radiation, the natural balance of my intestines was upset. This allowed a certain type of bacteria to grow out of control. It was why I was nauseated and had smelly diarrhea. (Not necessarily diarrhea since December, but certainly the nasty diarrhea of Saturday.)

The bug is called "C Diff," or Clostridium Difficile. Put simply, it's a germ that causes diarrhea. The classic symptoms are watery diarrhea, fever, loss of appetite, foul stool odor, nausea, belly pain and tenderness. Those most likely to grow the bugs are idiots like me taking lots of antibiotics. Being immune compromised is another count against you, as is cancer itself. The stuff I took to suppress heartburn probably contributed to its growth.

The Difficile part of the name isn't for the difficulty in getting the bug under control (it tends to be antibiotic resistant) but because researchers had trouble working with it in the lab when they first discovered it.

I wasn't alone in being buggy; C Diff is the most common cause of infectious diarrhea in hospitals and nursing homes. Yep, it is infectious—I could give it to others like a cold.

It spreads by spores that go from unwashed hands to something that someone else touches. The spores can hang around a door handle or light switch for weeks, waiting to crawl onto the next victim, so serious housecleaning was definitely called for.

The hospital was going to be fanatic about cleaning. I had to use just one of the changing rooms in the Radiation Center; no one else would use that room. Anything I touched had to be wiped down. If I used the bathroom, make sure they knew so housekeeping could come fumigate. The valets would have to wear gloves. What a pain.

One way to determine if your diarrhea might be C Diff is: how smelly is it? My C Diff infected diarrhea was knock-your-socks-off stinky.

To get rid of C Diff, you take another antibiotic, specifically, in my case, Flagyl. Fourteen days, three times a day of it. Early detection of the condition and aggressive management are the key factors to recovery.

To help Flagyl kill the nasty bugger, you have to be extra extra clean.

Wipe things with Clorox Wipes, wash your hands to death, wash your laundry in hot water. Diluted bleach is most effective for killing C Diff spores. Do not touch anything to your mouth that isn't certifiably clean, especially your hands.

A complete cleaning list, provided by the Radiation Center:

- Wash hands with soap and water (not those alcohol cleansers—they aren't strong enough to kill C Diff,) especially after using the bathroom, before preparing food, and before eating. Do it for at least 20 seconds, or two verses of "Happy Birthday to you," using lots of soap and getting deep into your fingernails and between fingers. Scrub! Don't forget the wrists. Rinse by letting the water run down to the fingertips, not up to the wrist. Use a paper towel to turn the faucet on and off.
- Only use towels once to dry hands—better, use paper towels.
- Wear disposable gloves to handle anything exposed to stool (feces, poop, number two,) urine (water, tinkle, number one) and wound drainage (blood, gore.) Wash hands fanatically afterward.
- Frequently clean anything you touch, not forgetting toilet handles, door handles, phones, keyboards and mice. Clorox wipes or water with bleach added (9 parts water to 1 part bleach) is best.
- Wash your sheets extra often. Use hot water, bleach, and high heat in the dryer.
- Do an extra good job washing dishes or use a dishwasher.
- Empty trash every day, both kitchen and bathroom.

I will add: use Cottonelle wipes. I did, and did not pass C Diff on. My guess is that the thickness of the wipes kept the spores from seeping through the cloth onto my hands. Just don't count on Cottonelle doing all the work. I didn't do a research study.

There were two more suggestions to treat my buggy body. Drink lots of fluids (wash the intestines?) and get some probiotics or active culture yogurt. The idea was to restore a proper balance in the intestines as quickly and smoothly as possible.

Avoid fruit as it can worsen diarrhea. Don't take Imodium or Pepto-Bismol—avoid over-the-counter preparations for diarrhea because they can actually make the infection worse.

Why does it matter? If C Diff gets bad enough, it can lead to serious inflammation of the colon and kill parts of your intestines. Then you have an operation to cut out those parts and have problems for the rest of your life. That life might not be very long if C Diff remains rampant; it can perforate your colon and kill you.

Don't minimize the danger. Rick and I ran into a couple we knew. She has C Diff and had been hospitalized several times. She almost died several times. The elderly father of another friend keeps getting kicked out of nursing homes. See, he has to wear a diaper and he has C Diff. No one wants to run the risk of spreading this antibiotic resistant bacteria and no one wants to perform extreme measures again and again, day in and day out, to avoid contamination.

Whether or not I ever got rid of the bacteria completely was up in the air. As long as I had no symptoms, I would not be retested for C Diff. Can't say that made a lot of sense, but that was the way it was. Evidently, some people have it in their intestines naturally. As long as it isn't high in number, you are okay.

When did I get it? Who knows, but I suspect that it began during the fifth chemo cycle or crept up on me when I started radiation.

So then I had my radiation treatment, me lying on the table feeling like a leper. After, I decided I would go to Janet's for lunch. If I was a leper, I had already been there as a leper. After that, I would go home and call the doctor.

At home, I needed to use the bathroom. Diarrhea, what else? Just as I was finishing, the phone rang. It was Dr. Sanatio. Yep, he was ordering antibiotic. Yep, I already needed to make an appointment to see him; I would do so. Yep, I would be a good girl and take the antibiotic as ordered.

I took two antibiotic pills and no longer had diarrhea, so it was working. I would take it the full fourteen days and bless the medical community for knowing how to deal with C Diff.

Saturday, May 12, 2012

How do you like that? I felt so good, I went to some garage sales looking for a dresser. Martha took hers when she moved, leaving us short of drawers. No, I didn't find one, but I was going to have to live with this dresser for the rest of my life. I was picky. I got tired, but it didn't kill me.

Let's pick apart that "I got tired," shall we? Some garage sales equaled three. The first one, I breezed through. The second, I browsed slowly, even though there was little of interest to me. The third I almost passed up, but stubbornness made me get out of the car and walk up the driveway. It was a short driveway and I could park right there; I wouldn't have stopped otherwise. Be glad I didn't find a dresser. I would never have gotten it into the car. I had a triple whammy on my energy level: chemo, radiation and C Diff. Who knows where one left off and another began?

People were very solicitous of me. I obviously had been sick; I obviously was not completely well. Several women came up to me and offered chairs, assistance, a glass of water. It reminded me of when I was 8 months pregnant and went to the Renaissance Festival. People were careful of me then. No one, absolutely no one, jostled my very pregnant body. This says nice things about the human race. We take care of our own when we need to.

Monday, May 14, 2012

Martha took us to dinner for Mother's Day. I didn't feel like Mother of the Century, but it was a nice dinner. Don't like my kids spending their money on me. I just like having my love for them acknowledged and returned.

The line where my breast meets the chest wall under my breast was red and a little sore. We had been putting Aquaphor there, but I decided it might be hindering rather than helping. Maybe it wasn't letting enough air get to the area. I left it off this one time.

Continued to use Aloe Vera. (I went through at least a 6 oz. tube each week.) I was smearing Aloe Vera on the red parts of my breast during the day, always at least once, and Rick was treating the whole breast nightly. He would put the Aloe Vera on and then wait for it to dry before smearing Aquaphor on the scar tissue and nipple area. One night I fell asleep while he was doing it.

Keep in mind that smearing means patting it on. Don't rub.

I didn't have a great deal of discomfort. My nipple itched sometimes. One day, I noticed that my nipple seemed inverted, but Mary told me it was probably that the areola (the colored area around the nipple) was swollen.

I felt energetic and normal. After radiation, I stopped at Moosejaw's to get Martha flip flops. Then I picked up a bottle of Probiotics.

These pills are marketed by various companies and sold alongside vitamins in the store. They contain good bacteria—good as in good for your colon and intestines. The Internet told me little about what C Diff does, but I did find a wealth of information about SIBO (Small Intestinal Bacterial Overgrowth,) when you have way more bacteria in your intestines than normal. I guess my bacterial infection qualified. The symptoms are the same: bloating, diarrhea and pain, along with excess gas.

The bacteria can interfere with the proper absorption of vitamins and minerals from food and can lead to weight loss. The recommended treatment is antibiotics (I was receiving the standard dosage for the standard length of time) and probiotics.

Probiotics have not received a lot of attention; there have only been a few studies done on them.

medicinenet.com says, "Commercially available probiotics such as VSL#3 or Flora-Q, mixtures of several different bacterial species, have been used for treating SIBO and IBS (Irritable Bowel Syndrome,) but their effectiveness is not known. Bifidobacterium infantis 35624 is the only probiotic demonstrated to be effective in treating patients with IBS."

(Be patient with all these impossible names, okay? I'll straighten it out by the end.)

Commonly sold probiotics might not be effective. They might not contain the bacteria listed on the label or the bacteria might be dead. Or they might have the wrong bacteria.

uptodate.com said S. boulardii, Lactococcus lactis, Lactobacillus rhamnosus GG, Bifidobacterium breve, and Streptococcus thermophiles are effective probiotics for C Diff. Lactobacillus rhamnosus GG was studied by the Cornell Medical Center and appeared to be especially good. Others said there wasn't enough evidence to support their use. When the experts can't agree, go with the ones who agree with your doctor. My doctor said to use probiotics, so I would.

Darn. The probiotics I bought had Lactobacillus gasseri KS-13, Bifidobacterium bifidum G9-1, and Bifidobacterium longum MM-2. I needed a bottle that had Lactobacillus rhamnosus GG.

In plain English, the bottle I bought had the wrong kind of bugs in it. I needed to go in search of Culturelle. Or Florastor. Or, if those two weren't available, DanActive. I should only shop in a reputable store because handling and storing these products badly can destroy the bugs in them. Heat kills living things, especially bacteria. Then they don't do any good.

Did you guess probiotics were not interchangeable? Live and learn. I took the pill I had purchased anyway, assuming that something was better than nothing, and promptly developed gas, the most common side effect of probiotics.

A gastroenterologist said you should take at least 5-10 billion CFU's (colony forming units) twice a day to benefit from probiotics. He also said probiotics stop doing good 2-4 weeks after you stop taking them, so I assumed I should be on them for at least a month to give my body time to get back to normal after I finished the antibiotic.

The other recommendation was to eat yogurt with active cultures. I don't like yogurt.

I spent a while on the computer, then lay on the bed to Aloe Vera my breast. Felt a little tired, so I closed my eyes and fell asleep. Woke up six hours later. Gassy.

Wednesday, May 16, 2012

Sharing a car isn't easy. I took Rick to the dentist and then he took me to my radiation appointment.

A crowd of "mucky mucks" were there. Henry Ford Health System was closing a location and they had a spare chemotherapist (as in the person who gives you a chemo treatment.) They were exploring the possibility of opening a chemo treatment center at Cottage Hospital. I wish they did it before I went through chemo; Cottage Hospital is so much more convenient to reach than Henry Ford Hospital. Less than half the driving time. Of course, it ran through the back of my mind that if I need chemo in the future...

I thought Rick would have to stay in the waiting room, but Mary invited him to hang out with us. He saw me on the table and got to stay with Mary while she ran the session from her control booth. She explained the procedure to him and he appreciated knowing more about what was happening to me. The only comment he made afterward was, "I watched your boob turn red again."

Thursday, May 17, 2012

In the afternoon, I had an appointment with Dr. Sanatio to go over the diabetic stuff. It's a long drive to Livonia, where he had been transferred, but I did it. He was too good a doctor—our relationship worked too well—to switch to another primary care physician.

I was worried. After starting the antibiotic and probiotic, my blood sugar soared. It was up and down, sometimes over 200, almost as high as it had been when I took the steroid. Dr. Sanatio still thought the diabetes thing was temporary. His guess was that the beating my body was taking with radiation and more medicine was manifested by the sugar. It should come down. Be patient.

I wanted to stop taking the blood pressure medicine, and he said I could try going without it. I did have to promise to monitor my pressure daily and report back to him in two weeks. And if my pressure didn't behave, go back on the Metoprolol. That blood pressure tester I didn't want to buy ended up being used more than I have would have thought.

Much as he would like to see me stop smoking, he wouldn't give me a prescription for Chantix, which was my only hope for quitting. Let the dust settle first, he said.

And finally, Dr. Sanatio showed me a picture of the kitten he was adopting. A long haired brown tabby with droopy ears, she looked like she belonged in a Cat Fancy centerfold. I was given the honor of naming her. Hereafter, let that sweet thing be known as Suzy Q.

Tuesday, May 22, 2012

My blood pressure and pulse became more erratic. Sometimes higher, sometimes lower. Nothing at a dangerous level, but definitely swinging. So I was off the Metoprolol for only a few days. I had to remember to let Dr. Sanatio know I was popping those pills again.

This was my last week of radiation, I thought. Dr. Solaris added an additional five days of treatment. He called it a boost. Beyond that, he was very pleased with the condition of my skin. I was so fair, my skin began reddening the first day, so he thought I would have problems. Mary said it was doing well because I was keeping it clean, and doing such a good job smearing Aloe Vera and Aquaphor on. Persistence can make a huge difference.

How did I keep it clean? I used my trusty Olay wet cleansing towelettes, the kind for sensitive skin. They aren't perfumed and don't have alcohol, just what the doctor ordered. Several times a day I wiped under my breasts, trying not to scrub, to mop up perspiration and dirt. I wasn't wearing bras and my heavy breasts sat on my stomach, getting stinky and sticky. Olay wipes were soothing, and if results mattered, remarkably effective at cleaning the skin without irritating it. Distilled water soaked into a well-worn cloth diaper (what's softer than an old diaper?) would be as good, I suppose. The most important thing was to dab, not scrub.

My breast was quite red now, with clear lines, especially on my stomach, showing where the radiation hit the skin. The underside of my breast, the seam where it meets the chest wall, was the least happy. It had turned purple, like a bruise, and the skin was hardened in a slight ridge.

It wasn't a bruise, it's the way radiation affects the skin, but it didn't feel good. Aside from random shooting pains that lasted less than a second, it was uncomfortable.

I was fortunate. Dr. Solaris told me if the skin broke down and seeped, I would be hospitalized, and that did not happen. They don't treat problems lightly, perhaps because radiated skin does not heal as quickly or as easily as un-radiated skin. It wouldn't do much good to be healed of cancer and die from icky skin.

I spent at least an hour every day, in sessions, flat on the bed with my skin uncovered to air it out. That seemed to do almost as well as Aloe Vera in soothing the seam. Also, I had not been using a pillow. The slight raising of my head on a pillow buried the seam in flesh and I wanted it exposed.

I was still on antibiotic for the bugs and diarrhea was a thing of the past. The stools were not firm, but they were getting there. I purchased Culturelle and took it daily. But I stuck my tongue out at Dr. Solaris and told him it was his fault. Over the weekend I had developed a bad taste in my mouth. One I was totally unable to describe. My mouth just tasted bad. And my tongue was coated.

"Not thrush," he said. He didn't know what it was.

Blame Culturelle. I decided not to take it for a few days and see what happened. And I was right. One day without the probiotics and my mouth tasted a little better. My tongue started to recover. So I decided I would wait until I finished the antibiotic before starting again with Culturelle—and maybe I would only take it every other day. Hindsight is 20/20: I should have suffered the icky mouth and kept up with Culturelle.

The receptionist said that the fatigue of radiation is similar to being out in the sun too long. You know the feeling; your arms are heavier, harder to lift and you just don't have the energy to do more than pop open a beer or pour water over ice cubes. As Grandma used to say, "Your get up and go got up and went."

The girlfriend of the valet at Cottage Hospital had lung cancer. She had her first chemo treatment and was promptly hospitalized because her platelets were so bad. She was sick as a dog, poor girl.

Friday, May 25, 2012

By Thursday night, the seam at the bottom of my breast had lost it. The thin layer of purple skin started to flake off, exposing red raw me. Lord almighty, did it sting.

By Friday morning, perhaps an inch of raw underside was exposed. When I went for my last full treatment, the doctor gave me Sulfadiazine cream and nonstick Telfa pads to tuck under my breast. Sulfadiazine was incredibly soothing; it took away the sting immediately. Looking it up on the Internet, it is an (expensive! It has silver in it. Look up the price of silver) antibacterial cream used to prevent and treat infection of second and third degree burns. Sulfadiazine's downside is it delays healing.

Aha! I had a radiation burn, although no one voiced the words. It's probably too scary a concept to introduce. When you realize that sunburn is also a burn, a radiation burn becomes less fearsome. They both hurt and both will heal. Sulfadiazine also works against yeast infections, I guess by passing good thoughts to the blood. Hallelujah. I still had a yeast infection under my breasts (I wasn't supposed to treat it and it was digging in happily) up close and personal with my raw strip.

The Telfa pads kept everything from sticking together.

I finished the antibiotic; let us hope the nasty bugs were dead in my intestines. As I promised, I started taking Culturelle again.

Monday, May 28, 2012

What an awful Memorial Day weekend. The raw strip under my breast widened to about 2½ inches, though it stayed very skinny. It made movement painful. It stung, it burned. It was almost as bad as a kidney stone or giving birth (both of which I have experienced.) Getting in and out of bed could bring on tears; just exposing it to air made me cringe. While Rick smeared Aloe Vera near the raw section, I kicked the bed and bitched.

I dug into the medicine cabinet and found some unused Tylenol with codeine. As long as I took it on a regular schedule, I could function.

Not that I did. Function, that is. The weather turned hot, which made me sweat, which wasn't pleasant for the underside of my breast. I spent hours lying on the bed half dressed, letting my sore boob breathe. I read books and slept. When I wasn't on the bed, I was in the living room in a chair, trying not to move. Holding my breast tightly when moving made it hurt less some of the time.

Grosse Pointe holds a community garage sale in the three story parking garage in the Village (a three block shopping district.) I didn't know if there was one this year. Didn't care about going, though it's lots of fun.

Saturday, my breast turned redder, which I had not thought possible. That was yesterday's radiation making its effects known. I was now itchy from under my armpit to the sternum, with the breast smack in the middle. It could be a sign that the skin was beginning to heal—or it could be a sign that my skin was on its last legs, I supposed. Whatever the cause, commonsense said "Do not scratch!" and I didn't. Lightly pressing on the site of an itch would make it subside for a while. I spent a lot of time pressing my fingertips in various places. Under my arm was the worst.

My nipple had looked inverted, indicating swelling. The breast felt too heavy when I lay down, sagging uncomfortably to the side.

I imagined a tight band around my chest roughly where the bottom of a bra would sit. Eileen said the tight band was a normal reaction to radiation, as was the swelling. (More about that tightness later. If you want to skip to it, look for where I talk about physical therapy and yoga.)

When Rick put Aloe Vera on Saturday night, my skin objected and got even scratchier. Sunday, I went without Aloe Vera for the day to give my skin some breathing space. I also went without the Sulfadiazine during the afternoon. The raw area began to dry, which made it sting less. But I wasn't sure if I was supposed to dry it or keep it moist, so Rick silverplated me later in the day.

I was also constipated. Whether it was a result of taking Tylenol with codeine or from the Culturelle, I didn't know. Two doses of Culturelle and the coating on my tongue began to return. Also the nasty taste in my mouth. I dug into a bag of Doritos, figuring the sheer bulk would help with the constipation. Wasn't it nice that the strong taste banished the slight distaste and some of the coating on my tongue.

No more Culturelle. It reminded me of chemo. (Bad girl.)

Tuesday, May 29, 2012

During the night, I dreamed that I needed to take a Tylenol. When I did wake up at 4 am, I was confused, unsure whether I had taken a pain pill or not. As a result, I did not take one, setting my sights on 8 am as a safe time for another dose. Let's not say I slept well.

I took a Tylenol at 8 am. That would have it at full dosage when I went for radiation. Nevertheless, raising my arm for treatment was painful. The doctor came to check my skin while I was on the table; it saved us having to lift my breast for examination later.

His instructions were to continue using Sulfadiazine and treat my skin as I had been doing. The raw slit should begin to feel better in 3-4 days. He wrote a prescription for Tylenol 3, thinking that Tylenol 4 was a possible cause of the constipation.

The nurse elaborated. The raw section would be better kept moist when I was dressed. It would not hurt to have it dry out; lie on the bed with it exposed all I liked, which would dry it out, but it should be moist if anything were to touch it, such as a Telfa pad or fabric. Once I was ready to sit up, I should pat Sulfadiazine on again. And continue to buffer the area with the nonstick Telfa pads so I didn't pull any newly forming skin off.

Thank God I was almost finished with radiation. I believe treatment would have been delayed until that nasty raw area healed if it was to receive more rays. As it was, treatment was seamless.

The Boost

Dr. Solaris had added an additional five days of treatment—doses to only the site where the tumors had been, not to the whole breast. He called it a boost. Mary assured me this extra treatment was now the standard of care, meaning it should be done unless there is a very good reason not to do it.

texasoncology.com says: "The European Organization for Research and Treatment of Cancer conducted a clinical trial evaluating 5,318 women diagnosed with stage I or II breast cancer who had undergone a lumpectomy followed by the standard dose of radiation. Approximately half of the patients were given an additional small dose of radiation (16 Gy) to the area where the cancer had been located, while the other half received no additional treatment. Data indicated an additional dose of radiation to the site of the removed cancer reduced the overall rate of a local recurrence by nearly 50%." The only drawback is a slightly higher risk of scarring.

As if another scar on my lumpectomied boob made any difference.

Now it was time for the boost of radiation.

I was in the accustomed position on the table, but the machinery made adjustments. It no longer swung around to my right side; everything happened on the left. The dose was targeted to about 5 o'clock on my breast (with the nipple as the center of the clock) in an area roughly the size of a racquetball ball. Mary told me it was not going deep into my breast; the area was quite near the skin. Attachments on the machine concentrated the "death ray." There was a long burst after which the therapists had to enter the room and change the attachment. I then received a second burst.

That is all there was to it. If the underseam of my breast had not become so upset, it would have been a speedy, uneventful visit. They did not anticipate any difficulties with the skin that was receiving extra radiation. Treat it with Aloe Vera as usual. And don't forget Aquaphor on the scars and nipple.

The constipation began to break up.

Monday, June 4, 2012

Today is the last day of radiation. The end of all treatment. What a strange feeling. I deserve a gold star; not once did I cancel an appointment. Every iota of treatment was accomplished without interruption, as the doctors wanted. I am the ideal patient. I managed to set myself up with the best possible chances to be cured. I am getting free of you, Cancer.

I had spent the last seven months concentrating on purifying my body, removing every last shred of cancer from my breast. After today, life should return to normal. I was no longer committed to a daily visit to Cottage Hospital. I wouldn't have a pressing reason to go near a medical facility. I wouldn't even see a doctor for a good six weeks unless I scheduled a visit. It was intimidating, this abrupt process of returning to normal.

Not to say I was done with all doctors and all cancer related matters. I would have mammograms every six months, probably until eternity. I needed to set up an appointment to follow up with the surgeon, though I had no intention of doing so. I couldn't see any point to it. Every month or six weeks I should get my chest port flushed. I had an appointment with chemotherapy oncologist Dr. Medica and there would be a follow-up appointment with radiation oncologist, Dr. Solaris. I should check with primary care Dr. Sanatio as to whether I needed a second test for the C Diff bacterial infection.

The overriding concern was the condition of my skin. Lordy, lordy, my breast looked terrible. And in a few very small spots, it felt badly. Overall, the skin was extremely red and mottled, as if I had wandered around Disneyworld for a week from 8 am to 8 pm with no sunblock, no shirt, no nothing to protect my skin. It was dry and itchy, but it did not hurt as if it was burned.

The closer you got to the nipple (Ground Zero in my imagination) the pores began to look dark, not with blackheads, but colored a deeper red than the skin. My nipple was somewhat sore. Also itchy. At least it was not swollen, or if it was swollen, it was not as noticeable as before.

The skin in the area that received the boosts had bagged, kind of like under your eyes. Rick had begun patting Aloe Vera on that spot, rather than spreading it, in case the skin decided it was going to tear off. It was a little more sensitive than the rest of my breast. Just close enough to be brushed by my arm; it hurt a teeny tiny bit.

There was a good amount of swelling on the outside of my breast; I laid it on a pillow so poor boobie didn't sag into my arm in bed. There was an uncomfortable feeling, like I had a ball inside my breast. I could push that ball around when I lay on my back. I again noticed bouncy bouncy when I walked.

Under my breast was still the troublesome area. The raw parts had begun to heal, but they still hurt like the devil. A second area on the underside of my breast had a flap of dead, black/purple skin hanging. It came loose over the weekend and I studiously did not pull it off. I was paranoid: so far, there wasn't any pain, but I couldn't be sure there wasn't a small bit of rawness there. Other sections of the purpled swash were coming loose. Hopefully, that was a natural sign of healing. I would check with the Radiation people. It was almost time to get dressed and go.

It was my last time through the wooden doors into the Radiation unit. Everyone met me like an old friend. My blood pressure was fine, no temperature. I was gifted with more Telfa pads, and I got hugs from everyone. Mary said she was sorry I was done; Eileen suggested ten more sessions so we could chat. I gave everyone the business card for my published books. These women were interested in my books, always a thrill to a writer. When the doctor came in, the first words out of her mouth were, "Why didn't I get a card?" She handed me my purse and I dug one out, warning, "They are romances." She didn't see anything wrong with light summer reading.

I had my orders. Keep using the medications, Aloe Vera and Aquaphor. Keep using Sulfadiazine and the nonstick pads on the raw parts. Expect significant healing in a week or ten days or two weeks.

If anything turned yellow or green or smelled bad, come in right away. That would be infection, the last thing my poor body needed to deal with. Come back August 7th for a follow-up visit. I should feel marvelous by then.

We had a mini-graduation ceremony. I got a certificate and an afghan knitted by one of the volunteers of Cottage Hospital. I didn't cry, but felt regret that I would never see these new friends again. (Untrue! I would be back at the beginning of August for the follow-up visit.)

I went home, my breast not feeling all that comfortable. As others had reported, I had a funny feeling, cutting myself off from medical attention so abruptly. It is an emotional jolt to go from serious medical care to nothing in one day. But I could get used to it.

Once I felt good again, I would love it.

Otherwise, things were shaping up. I now had the ghost of eyelashes. My eyebrows were growing. Did you know eyebrows grow quickly? One day I looked in the mirror and there was nothing there. The next day, you could see charcoal colored eyebrows. That was honest to God hair coming back, not fully enough to be dark haired eyebrows, but beginning.

The hair on my head was growing. It was just long enough that I did not feel like a total freak if I went without a covering. Saturday, Rick and I attended the opening of the congressman's campaign office, me in the glory of bareheadedness. I didn't notice any second glances. My hair was still white, but was getting a little silvery. No more flour head. I had hopes that, if it wasn't going to be dark, at least it would be a pretty white.

I should mention that the back of my head was not nearly so cooperative. Like a baby who fails to grow hair where her head rubs in the crib, the back of my head was not growing so well. But I didn't look at it, so what did I care?

My skin was still very dry, as were my sinuses. I drank a lot of water, feeling on the verge of dehydration. The skin on my face, especially my forehead and nose, still peeled easily as if the skin was more delicate. At the base of my thumbnails and a few of the other fingernails, normal nail was growing out of the bed. The sun was rising on the world; you could see a definite difference between dark and light. Yes, I would eventually have normal fingernails.

The neuropathy was disappearing. My fingers felt nearly normal; they almost never felt tingly or numb. Holding a needle was not as difficult. My feet still felt wrong, but that was lessening. My legs hadn't gone weak on me; I had no difficulty walking. Losing my breath was a thing of the past.

My bowels were more normal, although since finishing the antibiotic for the bacterial infection, they were slower than they used to be. Instead of a bowel movement every morning, I had one every two or three days. Was this an expected reaction to C Diff, or was I perhaps still infected?

My appetite was depressed. Again, was this C Diff's fault? Or some other problem? Or had I managed to shrink my stomach to nothing? Had my metabolism clicked into a higher gear or something?

Whatever the reason, I continued to lose weight—five pounds last week. I couldn't help but cheer. I could stand to lose much more than five pounds. The doctor would say that losing weight like that is never a reason to cheer.

My blood sugar was stabilizing and perhaps going into acceptable (non-diabetic) ranges. I thought. Hoped.

I still was troubled by whatever was coating my tongue. It affected my taste buds, though not to the extent mucositis had during chemo. It made my mouth dry. The doctor suggested brushing my tongue with a baking soda covered toothbrush.

I still got so tired. I needed naps. I could fall asleep at the drop of an eyelid. I didn't have energy. But I could feel it coming back.

I went to Meijer and bought new cat food bowls.

Dear Cancer,

You've about had it. I've done everything I should do; the doctors have added their much larger bits. I can't imagine that you kept a toehold inside me.

I have begun thinking that I am as fortunate as Mom and Lalie, that medical intervention beat you into the dust as it did their tumors. I wish I knew what type of breast cancer they fought, but I doubt medicine knew the difference between plain and triple negative tumors in the 1960's. They certainly didn't know about you in the 1920's.

The nicest thing to come out of my battle is I feel ever so much more connected to Mom, and that is saying a lot. We were always close. I am saddened that she had to go through Hell. I wish I had realized how hard it was for her. I wish I could have helped her more. She forgives me, I know.

She is sitting on a cloud in Heaven cursing you and cheering me on. Thank you, Mom.

See, now you've made me cry.

Tuesday, June 5, 2012

As the skin heals, the very dark radiated skin begins to slough off. The radiated skin rolled back like nylons down your leg, pushed by the friction of skin rubbing against skin (my saggy breast rubbing against my stomach.) The pink new skin exposed under it was outraged. I called it creeping blight. Radiation Nurse Jennifer said it was the experience burn patients go through, but as I had never suffered a burn to speak of rather than your garden variety sunburn, that told me nothing.

Don't peel the loose skin off; let it detach naturally. Allowing lukewarm water to flow over it in the shower will take off what is willing to come. No hot water, please, as the new skin under all that junk is very sensitive. Cold water is stupid.

Come prepared with your choice of pain reliever. Newly forming skin is sensitive. You are growing nerve endings and they overreact with displeasure at every movement. It stung. Stung. Stung. Hissing, kicking the bed, snapping at hubby stings.

I got it down to a system. Clean the breast ever so gently, then slather on Aloe Vera. Let it dry and then slather Aquaphor on the appropriate parts. On raw areas, spread Sulfadiazine until it stops stinging—more here, less there, keeping in mind that silver is hideously expensive and not to be wasted. Hiss and kick the bed until the stinging lessens.

It sometimes disappeared—thank you St. Agatha, patron saint of breast cancer sufferers, or was it St. John the Apostle, patron saint of burn victims?—but often enough, it still stung.

At that point, plaster a nonstick pad over the stings and sit up, swearing at having to move, which made it sting more. Sit still until everything calmed down, perhaps fifteen minutes if I had already popped a Tylenol 3.

Telfa pads under my sagging breast gave some measure of relief even when it didn't sting. The weather had turned hot and sweat made me uncomfortable. At least it didn't seem to add to the stinging. I had to change the pad every few hours because it would get slimy.

The drug store's brand of Telfa pads were thicker than those provided by Henry Ford and tended to slip more. They felt more irritating on uber sensitive skin. So I raided the pharmacy and found Curad nonstick pads. They were smaller (3x4 versus 3x8) and not quite as sturdy around the edges as Henry Ford's pads, but they felt much better tucked under my breast.

To compensate for size, I taped two together (overlapping) with masking tape, positioning the tape so it didn't touch my skin. I lay the pad along the seam of my breast so it folded when I stood up. (This is hard to describe!)

As the line of new skin crawled up my breast toward my nipple, I began taping a third pad on the top, pyramid wise, to keep the new skin protected. The whole idea was to keep any and all affected skin protected by a pad and to keep masking tape from touching me. If you have smaller breasts, you'll need less pad, but they will fall off. Big sagging breast held the pad in place.

Can you imagine wearing a bra under these circumstances? I didn't.

I gave up on handkerchiefs under my breast. They sopped up sweat nicely, but also ripped the new skin off once the Aquaphor and Sulfadiazine dried. Once the new skin turned a normal color, it was no longer very sensitive, but was more prone to chafing. It takes time to toughen up skin.

One area was extremely sensitive although the skin there was in relatively decent shape. It was the fold of breast that runs into the underarm at the bottom. There was a dark line of radiated skin, but around it was piercingly painful normal skin. Why that normal skin hurt/ached/itched so much was beyond understanding, but it did. While other parts of my skin toughened up, that area bothered me so much that I didn't like to have my arm brush against it. Alternatively, I would use a finger or two to push that area in; maybe I looked weird with my arm cocked, holding my side like I was staunching a gunshot wound, but I was beyond caring what I looked like.

No, this discomfort didn't surpass that of chemo, nor of the lumpectomy, but I was getting mighty tired of not feeling well.

Monday, June 11, 2012

I still had C Diff. Another round of antibiotics and despite the dull taste in my mouth, I started back on Culturelle. I had to kill the bugs.

I was more sensitive to the heat of summer. Air conditioning was not a luxury, but a necessity. I avoided the sun, as my skin did not like it, judging from the reaction of my forearms. That skin dried up and blew away from the sun. It also lost pigment in some areas, leaving me mottled.

This condition was not new for me—my left arm, which hangs out a car window all the time, had begun to mottle a couple of years before. It might be a condition called Vitiligo or it might just be a function of skin damage from too much sun. My much darker skinned brother has it on his back, so there might be a genetic component working here.

What was new was that with just casual time spent outside, my right arm did the same thing. Wham, bam. Mottled. I looked like a polka dot alligator. I took to smearing Aloe Vera on my arms, which helped smooth out the coloring and certainly helped with dryness, but bathing in Aloe Vera to recover from an extended period of sunbathing was laughable. The condition of my arms reminded me that chemo had done a job on my skin.

I had a touch more energy every day, but thanks to sore skin, even bending was awkward. My daughters paid for a cleaning service to clean my house. I guess they figured the dust balls were going to eat me and Rick. The house was cleaner than it has been since we moved here twenty some years ago. I still needed naps, perhaps not every day, but they were in clean rooms.

If my hair would grow, people might not realize I had spent months battling a serious illness.

Post-Treatment

Friday, June 22, 2012

If you doubt that lumpectomies, chemotherapy and radiation mess you up, banish those doubts. They pile on each other like football players and smother your efficiency. Or something.

Editing this book, I already knew I had mangled tenses (is it tomorrow or yesterday?) but I thought I fixed those mistakes. Wrong. There were a slew of is's to change to was's. Not only that, I lost whole entries somewhere. Huh? I typed them and failed to save them. This is unheard of for me, folks. I know how to save material. Didn't manage it. I goofed up a bunch of dates also. Not good. Thank God, I was over that.

This is chemo brain. I did not escape it. (Later, my daughter told me that it was clear to everyone else that I had been afflicted. I was the last to recognize it.)

Wednesday, October 17, 2012

We went to Sacramento in July. I used an umbrella at all times outside; my skin was sensitive to sun and Sacramento has more sun than anyone should live with. Yes, when my arm was exposed, it hurt. Kind of a crawly feeling, as if I was getting a sunburn, although my arm wasn't in the sun long enough to burn. But we had a marvelous time. I cuddled the cat Sibley, petted Arwen, who condescended to allow it, and enjoyed my semi-healthy self and Rick being with Katie.

Tap water was undrinkable in both Sacramento and Detroit. I couldn't even use ice cubes made with it.

Remember the Titanic exhibit I hoped to see? We went at the end of August. I was able to walk through it with no problem; I maneuvered through dense crowds okay. Enjoyed the exhibit, but saw no signs of ghosts.

We held a family reunion in August. It wore me out, but the girls did most of the work. I loved, loved, loved having my brothers and their families here. Afterward, I took lots of naps.

Still fighting C Diff. I was going to have a colonoscopy to do a stool transplant. Yes, it is just what it sounds like. They were going to plant some of my husband's stool in my colon. Gross, gross, gross, but it works. One clinical trial refers to the "Ick factor." I agree, but I needed to get rid of C Diff and this procedure is miraculously effective. At least I hadn't given it to my family. Hopefully no one in the world caught it from me.

Last time I used a bathroom at the hospital, there was a note taped to the wall. You don't need soap and hot water to wash C Diff bacteria off your hands. Rinsing in cold water is effective.

I had a dot on my back that was eczema and a patch on my elbow that was psoriasis. No prior history of either skin condition, so you know I blamed treatment. I instituted a moratorium on shaving my legs. My skin got irritated from a razor, and those areas turned into pinprick bits of eczema or psoriasis. Couldn't tell which, but the spots itched. I figured it was better to go hairy for the winter than to end up a blob of offensive skin.

I still got awfully tired, but it was no longer debilitating. I just vegged out when I got pooped.

Physical Therapy and Yoga

Found out that stretching was a critically important part of radiation recovery. What happens to cause that? The effects of radiation continue for months after you stop relaxing under the gray-grilled machine. One common side effect is a tightening of the muscles that bathed in the rays.

One very pertinent muscle for me was the serratus anterior—or was it the abdominal head of the pectoralis major—or maybe the external oblique muscle. Alternatively, it was the latissimus dorsi muscle. (Can you tell that I never verified what muscle it was with a doctor?) Whichever it is, the darn thing runs from under my breast around to my back. It started to stiffen up and it wanted to mess up my shoulder also. Things can get so tight that you lose mobility, as in your arm won't swing around properly. That was what I noticed first. My arm didn't go over my head easily.

Stretching can help limit that effect. Think of your body like Silly Putty and stretch in every direction.

The more technical explanation is that the muscles affected by radiation need to heal as much as the skin. But they tend to grow scar tissue. Think of a rubber band growing scars. When you stretch the rubber band, the scars pull. Mega ouch. Stretching those muscles will encourage the scar tissue to form in a less nasty manner. You have perhaps a six month window to worry about and ever after, you will be glad you made the effort.

The muscle under my radiation burn was tightening up. My arm wouldn't go over my head without discomfort. I contorted my torso, trying to keep that muscle stretched, without measurable success. I tried physical therapy. The therapist could not get the idea what I was attempting to do; he wanted me to strengthen all my muscles, front and back. My back muscles do not appreciate exercise because I have a bit of scoliosis (curvature of the spine) that damaged them. Short explanation is that I twanged certain back muscles too often over the years and they gave up. I learned years ago how to live with them, but the therapist's exercises irritated them rather than doing what needed doing, as in stretching front muscles. I gave up on therapy.

Then I found yoga. (Sounds like I fell in love, doesn't it? Didn't ride off into the sunset, so it wasn't love, just the right exercises for my underboob muscle.) Yoga stretches and strengthens muscles.

The position where you lay on the floor and swing your right leg over to the left (which twists your torso) was a dandy choice for keeping my bothersome muscle stretched. The pose is called the Supta Udkarshansana—Lying Abdominal Twist. You don't have to do this one perfectly, just enough to feel the stretch. Another pose that twanged my underboob misery was the cow pose, especially when I did it enthusiastically.

There may be a pose or two that works on your sad muscle. Consult a yoga teacher or look up poses on the Internet or in a book. Try a few; you may be surprised what ones catch hold of your scarring rubber band.

I had a PET scan which didn't show anything more than normal post-treatment changes. I had a mammogram which showed one or two clusters of microcalcifications midway between the two biopsy sites in my breast. The first biopsy (nearly a year ago) showed a cyst with a microcalcification or two; it all turned out to be two tumors, one DCIS and the other invasive, both triple negative. Now I had another biopsy scheduled. Please, God, not more cancer. But if it was... I would keep fighting. I'd rather go down with the ship than give up.

Do you hear that, Cancer? Not putting up with you anymore.

Sunday, April 27, 2014

The biopsy didn't show anything. The radiologist put me back on yearly mammograms. I objected, but was ignored. I was scared to just have them yearly, but then Dr. Medica ordered the chest port removed.

That felt like a vote of confidence in my health. Cancer free! What a thought. The removal was like the insertion, only in reverse, and recovery was much simpler. It felt good to get that tube out of the vein in my neck.

Eighteen months later, most of the aftereffects of cancer treatment were gone. My toes no longer hurt from neuropathy, although the same wasn't true of my fingers. Sometimes cold made my fingers ache, as in really ache. I may never clean snow off the car again without wearing gloves or carelessly handle ice cubes. Some days I had more trouble holding a sewing needle than others. On bad days, I could flip the needle out of my fingers. It would fly across the room. Watching it happen, I saw I was holding the needle in a death grip though I couldn't feel it as such.

I had trouble with paper. It was hard to turn a page. Typing was not effortless; it was hard to tell where my fingers were on the keyboard. I think my legs were pretty much better, but then again, at odd moments, they felt a little weak. I took up yoga and was amazed how my legs shook, but they didn't collapse.

I used to have nice eyebrows. I used to have eyelashes. Didn't have a full crop anymore. No one warned me that eyelashes and eyebrows could (and did) fall out on a regular basis. I'd be clomping along just fine and would suddenly enter shedding season. Couldn't find a rhyme or reason for it. It just happened.

My hair was the pits. It wasn't growing well yet, but please note the "yet." It was growing and I was confident it would continue to improve. I grew hair on the nape of my neck and vaguely in the sideburn area; it was baby fine and curled unevenly. This spring, my hair started to get greasy. You know, when you don't wash it enough and you sprout an oil slick? Finally happening.

My skin looked old. Nothing helped, so I resorted to prayer. Maybe better health would result in better skin. Still, it's a lot better to look old than to look dead.

My blood sugar went to normal and I threw away the diabetic supplies. My cholesterol was through the roof, so my primary care physician put me on Gemfibrozil, which did a wonderful job pulling my cholesterol numbers into acceptable range, but it also threw my blood sugar off again. I was back on insulin and taking a different cholesterol lowering medicine, Pravastatin. Pravastatin is said not to mess with blood sugar. Cross your fingers that I eventually got these hobgoblins settled.

Since I had not succeeded in getting rid of Hydrochlorothiazide, the blood pressure diuretic, I knew my system had not fully recovered from chemotherapy. By the way, Hydrochlorothiazide can make you diabetic.

How fun.

I thought I escaped chemo brain, but I lied. It taunted me. Sometimes I was fine. Other times, I couldn't concentrate. I'd forget words. Typing could be a nightmare. I glanced at the monitor and saw I typed "rite" instead of "right." "Their" instead of "there." "Et" instead of "get." Tried to say "discourteous" and it came out uncourteous. Then incourteous. Had forgotten the word was discourteous. I was afraid to start a new novel. It's not the easiest thing to do, to write a book worthy of publication, and I was scared that I couldn't pull together a plot, much less find words to fill the plot out. I always included humor in my writing. That seemed lost.

Think of chemo brain as a nasty version of the mind you get when you go into menopause. You forget things. Words! What would I give to be able to pop out the right word? I knew the definition, how I wanted to use it, but I couldn't come up with the word. Watching Jeopardy was torture. I knew the answer, I knew I knew the answer! But I couldn't produce it.

I couldn't concentrate—I zoned out, couldn't pay attention. Oh, to be able to follow a conversation for more than a few minutes. I felt like the quintessential brainless blonde.

I noticed one very curious thing about my version of chemo brain. Being a writer, I need to dream up plots, but when I tried, my brain would freeze. I could feel it stop, stutter, try to figure out how to do it, and fail. Stop. Give up. It was as if I lost that ability. Except, I still had it. Just like the Jeopardy answer, I knew it was in there, it just wasn't getting out.

Stumbling blocks. I'd get over them. My days felt empty because I had not been writing.

Over time, my chemo brain improved. I worked through it. They say that chemo brain can resolve itself 18 months after treatment. I agreed. It wasn't as bad as it was before. I had far fewer bad days but it wasn't fixed completely yet. I decided to give it a little more time and if it didn't resolve, I would ask for help. Yes, there are things to be done medically to help chemo brain.

I didn't have many lasting effects from radiation. Darkening of the skin under my breast looked funny, since it's in a straight line, as if I laid a board over my stomach before I got a tan.

The muscle that runs under my breast got tangled up with scars and sometimes twanged. Tilting my torso just so helped. Pressing on the cramp generally made it behave, but when it didn't, the cramp wandered around to my back where it squeezed a rib.

I tried a couple different muscle relaxants to ease that muscle, but they didn't have much effect. A rum and Coke did wonders—but booze is not a wise way to medicate yourself. Danger, Will Robinson, danger! Drinking can do more damage than good. I'm not sure there is a simple answer to that muscle pain. Avoidance of the problem is preferable. I did do a good enough job stretching that my arm had full mobility. It no longer hurt to put it over my head.

I had more episodes of heartburn than before chemo. I carried antacids in my purse. It paid to be prepared. More importantly, C Diff was eradicated by the colonoscopy procedure.

Sadly, I gained twenty pounds. Much of that was because, being a good American, I couldn't keep my stomach shrunk. It stretched. My husband was content with the weight gain; he hated seeing me eat like a bird. I wished I could lose those twenty pounds and more, but couldn't resist yummy food.

Remember the casseroles I froze before I had the lumpectomy? I cleaned out the freezer in the basement and found a number of them. They went straight into the garbage. I also cleaned out my pantry, finding long expired foods. Please note it took me that long to realize I needed to purge.

I did wean myself off soda pop. I preferred water these days. I had to have bottled water—the stuff out of the tap had a funny taste. First, I was able to add ice cubes made from tap water, then I could actually drink tap water. Usually. Sometimes. My taste buds were still a tiny bit wacko. And bottled water felt safest.

Keep in mind that if you aren't drinking tap water, you are not getting fluoride, which is good for your teeth. You can buy a mouthwash that has fluoride in it to help make up the difference. Then you have to remember to use the mouthwash. Use toothpaste with fluoride.

The psychological effect of food concerns during treatment stayed with me. I'd look at meat that had been in the refrigerator two days and couldn't eat it. It had to be fresh. I was not interested in prepared products full of preservatives. I was more willing to cook from scratch to avoid chemically slick innards.

I was getting there. I felt healthier and had more energy.

To be honest, I felt more like a treatment survivor than a cancer survivor. But I was a survivor.

Monday, June 1, 2015

Happy three year anniversary. Three years cancer free.

Before my latest visit with Dr. Medica (in April,) I dreamed that I had cancer again. In the dream, I wasn't so upset about the cancer, but the thought of doing chemo again made me shiver. That was my first and only dream ever about cancer.

Let me do a quick runthrough of things that have not gone back to normal after three years.

- Still have neuropathy. My toes and feet are basically okay, though I sometimes have trouble going down stairs. It's as if I am not sure where my foot is on the tread. I have developed calluses by my toes, so I am walking differently. That could cause problems down the road. My fingers are sometimes a little numb. They are weaker (both hands are weaker.) Sometimes worse, sometimes better. Have lost some coordination: you know how you can twirl a pencil around in your hand to use the eraser? Sometimes I can't, sometimes I can. Every once in a while I will have a bit of trouble with my thighs, but not often. Occasionally I drool a little.
- I could use an eyelash and eyebrow transplant. They just never came back fully.
- If some people grow thicker, curly, luxuriant hair after chemo, you couldn't prove it by me. I do have hair, but it is thinner than it used to be and not quite that pretty silver. I have to wash it more often than pre-cancer or it goes limp. Periodically, I still shed what seems like an excessive amount.
- My skin is very dry. I have a lonely spot of eczema on my back and I wonder if I will ever get rid of psoriasis. My elbows are afflicted, as are the back of my head and neck. I get dots of it on my right hand and on my legs, but those come and go. Both skin conditions are related to the immune system and inflammation. My skin is sensitive—Cottonelle wipes are still my friend. Without them, I get the occasional hemorrhoid.
- Chemo brain is almost gone, though at odd moments, I forget words. I have trouble with plotting scenes, much less full stories. Watching an episode of Brain Games on TV, it seems to be a problem with communication between the right and left sides of my brain. I am thinking of seeing a neurologist. Shrink my head, please.
- Have problems with my blood pressure and retaining water. I still have diabetes, but am pretty sure (read hopeful) that I will beat it. (See the next entry.)
- My sinus problems are harder to control. Before treatment, I knew how to manage them when they acted up. Now, I seem to have less ability to stave off flare-ups. Last summer, I was on antibiotic for six weeks to try to cure it. It almost worked. What was curious

was that while the sinuses were almost fine, my blood sugar went normal. A specialist now thinks the problem is inflammation; medication, diet, and good karma might fix things. That is something I am actively working on. Have to get healed.

- I never quite got my stamina back. I still tire easily and have trouble sleeping through the night. Some or all of this could be the fault of my sinuses.
- My taste buds are okay, but Detroit water still doesn't taste right. I buy Aquafina (bottled water,) though I think I should be able to go without it. I can drink soda pop, but usually don't want it. I often feel like I am getting dehydrated and drink more water than I ever have in my life.
- I am less tolerant of hot and cold. Nothing dreadful, I just don't handle extremes of temperature as well as I used to.

That is about it. Not a bad list, right? I'll choose these irritations over cancer any day.

Cancer Antigens

After the visit to the oncologist, I had a blood test, checking for cancer markers. Did you know there is a whole religion centered on those numbers? Some doctors check them every couple of months. Some people panic or agonize over them. Others adopt a fatalistic view. I didn't even remember what they were.

Okay, let's explain cancer markers.

Early in my treatment, Dr. Medica tested my blood for cancer markers. We didn't go into the subject in detail, but she told me she wanted those results—the numbers—to compare later, to see if cancer had invaded me again.

The markers she tested are Cancer Antigen 27.29 and Cancer Antigen 15-3.

As the Dr. Susan Love Research Foundation says of 27.29, "It is the first and only blood test that is specific to breast cancer. (The two other blood tests that oncologists may recommend for women with breast cancer, the CA 15-3 and the CEA, are tumor marker tests that are used in breast and other cancers.) The CA 27.29 test measures the level of CA 27.29 antigen, which is found in the blood of breast cancer patients. As breast cancer progresses, the level of CA 27.29 antigen in the blood rises. In theory, by monitoring CA 27.29 test results oncologists can determine if the cancer has spread to other parts of the body..."

But the 27.29 test is not very accurate. It is not reliable and it isn't sensitive enough. So it is a guideline, not an absolute truth. Same thing with 15-3. But these tests are what the medical community have to guess if breast cancer is coming back. Of course they use them. Something is better than nothing.

Reading in Internet chat rooms, test results fluctuate. Get tested a bunch of times and your numbers float around. Results over 80 are bad, over 100 are bad, bad, bad. There were a few people currently battling breast cancer with numbers in the thousands; they used the tests as a guide to how well their treatment was progressing.

My results were:

	2012	2014	2015
CA 27.29	27.4	37.7	50.6
		good results are less than 38.6	
CA 15-3	21.7	22.8	23.8
		good results are less than 32.4	

Dr. Medica told me the 2015 test for CA 27.29 seemed flawed; all of her patients had elevated numbers. I should not worry about it. What, me worry? Of course, I worried, and still do. Those numbers are creeping upward, which might be a bad sign.

She slid my body through another MRI, which I passed with flying colors. No sign of cancer anywhere. Did it make me feel better? Yes, but not just because of antigens. It was nice to know that so far, I am cancer free. I don't intend to go into a funk over antigens, now or in the future.

Maybe a better test is coming. WebMD told me about a new blood test called cMethDNA that can predict whether cancer is going to come back. Wow. The test isn't available yet; I have to wait five years before I can take it, if then. They have to test it, refine it, make it more reliable. My vote is for immediate implementation—if the cancer marker tests currently in use are flawed, another that is also flawed is better than nothing.

Anyway, I applaud the Sidney Kimmel Comprehensive Cancer Center at Johns Hopkins University School of Medicine in Baltimore. That is the group working on cMethDNA.

What the test does is look at circulating tumor DNA in the blood. Does it contain any of ten breast cancer specific genes? Have they undergone a process called hypermethylation? If yes, evidently your cancer is alive and kicking. The test is not 100% accurate, but the idea of taking it made my stomach ping and summersault.

Dr. Joanne Mortimer, director of Women's Cancer Programs at the City of Hope Comprehensive Cancer Center in Duarte, California, said the worst part of being treated for early stage breast cancer is the period after treatment is over. "Then they [patients] live with this uncertainty. They may be cured, they may not. And only time will tell." She is so right. It is unsettling to not know.

The scary thing about triple negative breast cancer is that it seems to come back easier than other types of cancer. A Canadian study found that women with triple negative were at higher risk of having the cancer recur outside the breast, but only for the first three years after treatment. The longer you go without having it pop up, the less likely it is to do so.

Five year survival rates are lower with triple negative breast cancer. It doesn't seem to matter what stage you are when they catch it—treatment is less effective and more women die within five years than with other types of breast cancer. The good news is that all equalizes after the magic five year time period.

Not to say that the stage of your tumor doesn't matter; of course it does, especially with triple negative tumors. The sooner you find that nasty weed growing in your breast garden and chop it out, the less chance it has of blooming and sending seeds flying.

Has anything changed in breast cancer treatment since the 1960's? My answer is yes and no. The basic procedures for getting tumors out of your breast haven't changed.

The surgeon still has his day, but his scalpel will be much less destructive than it once was. He doesn't slice and dice; instead he has a very detailed plan to remove what must be removed and no more. Your body can certainly look better when he is done than it used to.

Oncologists still throw patients in the path of a radiation machine, but now that machine is computerized. It is capable of a delicate procedure which can avoid things like burning holes in your body that don't heal. They can even minimize the effects of radiation on your nipple.

They did chemotherapy in the 1960's—in fact they have been doing it since WWII (mustard gas gave scientists the idea it could be useful) but today there are new drugs and new methods of delivering those drugs. Add all the breakthroughs on handling side effects and you start to see vast improvements since the 60's.

Compared to the treatment my mother underwent, we are living in a brave new world. It's a lot more scientific and it will continue to improve via research and those pesky clinical trials. Eventually, doctors might reliably and consistently cure triple negative breast cancer. Wouldn't that be nice?

breastcancer.org says: "...new treatments such as PARP inhibitors are showing promise. Researchers are paying a great deal of attention to triple-negative breast cancer and working to find new and better ways to treat it."

"This is an exceptionally hot area of research in the breast cancer field," said George Sledge, MD, oncologist and member of the breastcancer.org Professional Advisory Board. "There is immense interest among drug developers, pharmaceutical companies, and breast cancer laboratory researchers in finding targeted therapies for these patients."

I am grateful for their concern and attention. Good luck!

Back when I first met breast cancer, research told me to be fatalistic and expect my cancer to recur within two years. If it missed that anniversary, I could start to breathe deeper, but I had to wait until my fifth anniversary to decide if I had been cured of cancer. What date is your anniversary date? It is the date you complete treatment.

To make it easy to remember, I set mine as June 1. In 2017 I will reach the magic five year mark. That's an awfully long time to wait for anything, but especially to wait for something to try to kill me. I could get downright neurotic. What if I consciously tabled all important plans until 2017? What if I unconsciously took that date into consideration? I could twiddle my life away.

The answer to this is vigilance. If you don't want to be overgrown with triple negative breast cancer, then you have to deal with it ruthlessly. Don't relax after you finish treatment. Get yourself to the doctor for any and all testing your insurance will cover. A yearly MRI sounds like a wonderful idea, doesn't it? But you also have to learn to live without constant medical attention.

Be strong. Get as healthy as you can. Eat a low fat diet. Have your mammograms done on time. Fight.

Do I want to hang around, with a gnawing feeling in the pit of my stomach, praying that cancer doesn't come back? I could do that, but I don't want to. I am trying to live my life as I lived it before I was diagnosed with triple negative breast cancer. I skimp on housekeeping, love my family, write, and enjoy myself. Thank God I've gotten over the fear of dying. I think it dissolved in the endless details of keeping healthy under bombardment.

I survived the important stuff: surgery, chemotherapy, radiation. I stayed sane and achieved clear mammograms and MRIs.

I told Eileen there isn't anything in my breast. I feel in my soul that there isn't anything there.

So pooh on you, Mr. Triple Negative Breast Cancer. I win.

I am a cancer survivor and life is good.

INDEX to side effects and symptoms
(definitions and significant discussions)

A
abdominal pain	85
ache or pain	16, 45, 62-3, 73, 85, 90, 92, 96, 98, 106, 141-2, 156, 160, 161, 171, 174, 188-9, 208, 214, *see also neuropathy*
acid reflux	*see heartburn*
acne	87, 91, 97
allergic reaction	61, 90
anemia	144, 161
armpit discomfort	50, 188, 202
arthralgias	*see ache or pain*
arthritis	107

B
balance	94, 142
Beau's lines	125
bleeding	62, 86-7, 107, 115-6
blisters	63, 97
bloating	156, 160, *see also water retention*
blood clots	50, 70, 77, 142
blood pressure	118
blurred vision	85
bone problems	16, 90, 106-7, 181, *see also ache or pain*
breathing difficulties	61, 63, 90, 119, 143, 156, 160-1, 188
bruising	62, 143

C
cataracts	*see eye problems*
chemo brain	211, 215
chest pain	63, 161, 188
chills	62, 106, 128, 160
cold sweat	88, 128, 142
confusion	142, 156
congestion	92
constipation	62, 85, 90, 92, 101-2, 156
coordination	85
cough	160
cramps	62, 92, 151, 156

D-E	dehydration	83, 95, 155-7
	depression	144, 156
	diabetes	118, 135-6, 159
	diarrhea	62, 85, 92, 156
	dizziness	63, 92, 142, 156-7, 161
	drooling	*see mucositis*
	dry mouth	85, 119-20, 134, 156
	dry skin	97, 156
	Dyspnea	160-1
	ears ringing	*see tinnitus*
	electrolyte imbalance	151
	eye problems	62, 67, 85, 130, 161
F-G	fatigue	85, 123-5, 143-4, 156, 160-1, 188
	fever	62, 106, 160
	fingernails	*see nails*
	folliculitis	*see hair*
	foot problems	141
	gas	84, 92
	glaucoma	*see eye problems*
H	hair	24, 62, 87, 92, 171, 188
	Hand-Foot Syndrome	*see foot problems*
	headache	90, 106, 142, 160-1
	heart problems	63, 124, 142, 151, 156, 160-1, 167, 188
	heartburn	139
	hemorrhoids	83
	hives	61, 97
	hot flashes	128
	Hyperglycemia	118
	hyperpigmentation	97
	Hypocalcemia	151, *see also electrolyte imbalance*
I	insomnia	*see fatigue*
	intestinal blockage	62, 101
	irritability	156
	itching	48, 61, 87, 98
K-M	Ketoacidosis	119
	Leukocytosis	167
	lips blue	156
	lips burning	*see mucositis*

	Lymphedema	56-7
	metallic taste	84, 150, 154, 169
	Mondor's Disease	50
	mouth	*see mucositis*
	mucositis	87-8, 101, 149
	muscle ache or pain	*see ache or pain*
	muscles tight	202-3, 212-3
	muscles weakening	*see neuropathy*
N	nails	96, 107, 125
	narrowing of tear ducts	*see eye problems*
	nausea	29, 62, 90, 93, 119, 156, 188, 192
	neuropathy	62, 101-2, 134, 162
	Neutropenic fever	156
	night sweats	*see hot flashes*
	nipple problems	69, 187, 197
	nose problems	105-6, 127
	numbness	47, 142, 151
		see also neuropathy
P-R	Palmar-Plantar Erythrodysesthesia	141
	perforation	77, 92
	peripheral neuropathy	*see neuropathy*
	photosensitivity	97
	pimples	*see acne*
	plaque (teeth)	169
	prominent veins	142
	psoriasis	97
	purpura	97
	radiation burn	201-2, 208
	red spots on skin	62, 106
	redness	87, 141
	rupture of the spleen	90
S	saliva	92
	sensitivity to sun	97
	shortness of breath	*see breathing difficulties*
	Sickle Cell Anemia	90
	side effects (anti-nausea drugs)	85
	side effects (biopsy)	8, 32
	side effects, dire (chemotherapy)	61-2
	side effects (lumpectomy)	48, 69

	side effects (Neulasta)	90
	side effects (port)	70-1
	side effects (radiation)	187-8
	skin discoloration	142
	skin pale	161
	sleepiness	156
	sleeping difficulties	49, 188, *see also fatigue*
	Steven Johnson Syndrome	97
	swallowing	87, 123, 156
	swelling	7, 57, 61, 63, 70, 80, 87, 106, 142, 187, 189, 202, 205
T-U	temperature	98, 110
	thrombophlebitis	50
	thrush	*see mucositis*
	tics and twitches	151-2
	tingling	87, 151, *see also neuropathy*
	tinnitus	92
	tiredness	*see fatigue*
	toenails	*see nails*
	tongue problems	87-9, 95, 117
	urination problems	62, 118
V-W	vaginal bleeding/dryness	86
	Vitiligo	210
	vomiting	*see nausea*
	water retention	62, 160
	weakness	62, 90, 95, 101, 131, 142, 156, 161, *see also neuropathy*
	weight gain or loss	61, 63, 94, 189
	wound healing	62

About the Author

Ann Tracy Marr, a novelist and computer consultant, admits to being sixtyish. Despite having published books, which many people think is exotic, she considered herself an average person living an average life.

Then, following in the footsteps of three generations of her family, Marr was diagnosed with breast cancer. Things changed.

She became the average cancer patient.

The diagnosis tightened. It was triple negative breast cancer. She was no longer average, but a high risk cancer patient.

To maintain her sanity, keep track of what was happening, and figure out what was going to happen, Marr acted like a typical writer and kept a diary of her thoughts, experiences, and research.

Now she is a Cancer Survivor.

Once her head was above water, Marr realized that others could benefit from the endless hours she spent researching surgery, chemotherapy, radiation treatment and the associated drugs and side effects. Her personal experiences may also be of value, if only as comic relief.

She hopes DEAR CANCER helps the reader gain insight, strength, and wisdom in dealing with cancer.

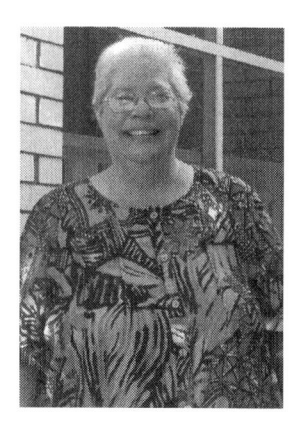

Other books by this author

A fantasy Regency romance series

Round Table Magician

Thwarting Magic

To His Mistress

available in ebook and paperback

...bright and fun and everything Regency...
Maura Frankman, The Romance Studio

...you will find yourself going back and forth over and over again thinking you have it figured out, only to find, you might not...
Angi, Night Owl Romance

...Those who feared that the Regency genre might be dead need not worry. It is kept alive and healthy by such authors as this who employ their fertile imaginations to reinvent the world...
Amanda Kilgore, eternalnight.co.uk

Connect with the author

at her webpage
http://www.atmarr.com/dearcancer.htm

on Facebook
https://www.facebook.com/anntracymarr

on Goodreads
https://www.goodreads.com/author/show/1146028.Ann_Tracy_Marr

on YouTube
https://www.youtube.com/user/marr794

for fun she is furnishing her Regency inspired house at
https://www.pinterest.com/anntracymarr/the-english-regency-inspired-house

email her at
anntracymarr@aol.com

Printed in Poland
by Amazon Fulfillment
Poland Sp. z o.o., Wrocław